ISBN: 9781077063570

Note: At publication, the off-the-shelf foods used in this book were widely available in most supermarkets. But food products come and go. So if there is a frozen entrée or soup selection in this diet that is out of stock, or that's been discontinued, or perhaps you don't like, or that you forgot to pick up while shopping, please substitute another food that has **approximately** the same caloric value and nutritional content. In this regard, many dieters have found the foods listed in the Appendices at the end of this book to be very helpful.

100-DAY

NO COOKING
DIET
1500-Calorie

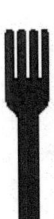

Elena Novak

NoPaperPress

CONTENTS

Too Busy to Cook?

Most of us are busy – extremely busy struggling to balance career, family, finances, and then you need to make room for a personal life, for friends, for learning, for travel and the list goes on and on. Because you're so busy, you may neglect your health. You know you should lose weight. You want to lose weight but don't have the time to cook and diet! Your life is just too hectic to plan and prepare elaborate low-calorie meals. This is where the *100-Day No-Cooking Diet* can help. A sensible, healthy weight loss diet with no cooking!

The Best Weight-Loss Diets

According to the late nutritionist Dr Jean Mayer, of Tufts University Department of Nutrition, every good weight-loss diet should have the following three characteristics:

1) A good diet must provide you with an understanding of weight control as well as the knowledge you need to lose weight.

2) A good diet must help you remain healthy while you are losing weight.

3) A good diet must lead you to a healthier way of eating and exercising that will, in the long term, help you keep off the weight you have lost.

The weight-loss diet featured in this book is the so-called "balanced diet;" i.e., a diet that is not only low calorie and reasonably low in fat, but is also nutritionally balanced . The *100-Day No-Cooking Diet*, however, does not meet all the criteria set forth above. While you will get some "dieting insight" and some idea of how much you can eat and still lose weight, you will not get a real understanding of weight control from this book. That's not its purpose. What you do get is a reasonably healthy diet – and a diet that if followed will promote weight loss, but it's not the long-term answer.

Long-term success is not about finding the "right" diet. It's about developing both an understanding and a plan that will result in healthier eating and physical activity habits. Without a doubt identifying the behaviors that have contributed to your eating more calories than your body needs is important, very important. But assuming you are successful in determining why you overeat, what do you do next? The truth is that weight control, although a relatively complex issue, is governed by a set of logical, scientific principles, and the acceptance and understanding of these principles – augmented of course by desire and self-discipline – can lead you to sure and lasting weight management. For a complete weight control discussion, a through understanding and the guidance you need to succeed we recommend you read, *Weight Control - U.S. Edition* by Vincent Antonetti, Ph.D., published by NoPaperPress.com.

Why a 90-Day Diet?

Experts agree that a diet that promotes weight loss over a relatively longer time period is healthier and the weight loss is likely to be more permanent. These experts recommend you choose a nutritious diet that results in a weight loss of approximately 2 pounds per week – which amounts to about 28 lbs in 100 days. The *100-Day No-Cooking Diet* fits the bill!

Before you begin any weight loss program you should **medical assessment, or exam.** Why? You need to make sure your health will allow you to lower your caloric intake and increase your physical activity. The physician conducting the medical exam should be made aware of and should approve the specific weight loss diet you're planning. In particular, you should **let your physician know that the *100-Day No-Cooking Diet* relies to a considerable degree on commercially processed convenience foods (frozen and microwaveable) – most of which have a relatively high salt (sodium) content**. Additionally, if you are going to engage in some sort of physical activity in conjunction with this diet and especially if you have been totally inactive, or if you have or suspect you have cardiovascular disease or other health problems, or if you are obese, or if you are 40 or older, before embarking on the physical fitness portion of your weight control program you should have a stress test supervised by a physician.

1500-Calories Right for You?

Most adults can and do lose weight on *100-Day No-Cooking Diet - 1200 Calorie Edition*. But how fast you lose weight is strongly dependent on the diet calorie level you choose. Okay, which diet calorie level should you choose?

- 1200-Calorie Diets are appropriate for most women – but are also effective for smaller men, older men and inactive men. (See *100-Day No-Cooking Diet - 1200 Calorie* also published by NoPaperPress.com.)

- 1500-Calorie Diets are suitable for most men – but are also effective for larger women, younger women and active women.

How Much Will You Lose?

Adults on any weight-loss diet invariably want to know how much weight they will lose – and how fast. Weight loss occurs when your food energy intake is less than the total energy you expend. This difference in calories is referred to as your <u>calorie deficit</u>.

How much weight you lose depends on the magnitude of your calorie deficit. Physiologists have long known that to lose one pound requires a deficit of approximately 3,500 Calories. Therefore, if a person's total calorie deficit over time is known, their weight loss over time can be calculated.

On the *100-Day No-Cooking Diet – 1500 Calorie*, **most overweight women lose 20 to 30 pounds.** Smaller women, older women and less active women will lose a tad less and larger women, younger women and more active women somewhat more.

On the *100-Day No-Cooking Diet - 1500 Calorie*, **most overweight men lose 30 to 40 pounds.** Smaller men, older men and less active men will lose a bit less and larger men, younger men and more active men usually lose much more.

Exactly how much weight you will lose is a bit more complicated and depends on how much you weigh, your gender, your age and your activity level. Again, for the full story see *Weight Control - U.S. Edition* by Vincent Antonetti, Ph.D.

Using the Daily Menus

Let's look at the **Daily Menu for Day 1** on page 16. Most of the menu is obvious and easily understood. Find the line item **Soup (see Appendix B on page 118)**, and note the soup calorie allowance is 110 Calories. Now go to **Appendix B** on page 118, which contains a list of 25 soup selections arranged from lowest to highest in calorie content. In Appendix B, scroll down until you find the 110 Calorie soup selections. There are two to choose from.

Now let's move on to **Day 2** on page 17. To find the frozen entrée for Day 2 first note that the allotment for the Day 2 frozen entrée is 290 Calories. Now go to **Appendix D** on page 122, which contains a list of frozen entrées arranged from lowest to highest calorie content. In Appendix D, scroll down until you find the 200 Calorie frozen entrées. There are lots of entrées to choose from.

Breakfast Guidelines

You've heard it before. It's important to start the day right and eat breakfast. **So try to allow time for breakfast before you rush off to work.** If need be do some preliminary preparation the night before such as setting up your coffee maker, deciding on and measuring the amount of cereal you will be eating, etc. Many busy people prepare breakfast at home and bring it to work in a plastic container. Do what you need to do – but don't skip breakfast!

When on the *100-Day No-Cooking Diet*, you may substitute any cereal specified for any other wholesome **whole-grain cereal**. For example, if you're not crazy about having Shredded Wheat for breakfast on Day 6, substitute Wheat Chex or Cheerios, etc. If you don't have the time to cook oatmeal on Day 7, substitute Wheaties. (Incidentally, you can make great tasting oatmeal in your microwave in about 1½ minutes.) And if you don't

like the soft-boiled egg called for on Day 10, have a hard-boiled egg or make a scrambled egg instead. Maybe the cantaloupe on the meal plan is not in season. No problem. Just replace the cantaloupe with a half cup of orange juice. A more complete list of food substitutions and exchanges can be found in **Appendix A** on page 116.

Lunch Guidelines

On most days of the *100-Day No-Cooking Diet*, lunch will call for either soup or a sandwich. For your convenience, soup choices have been limited to those sold in a microwaveable bowl. In fact, unless otherwise stated, assume the soups specified in the 90-Day meal plans are microwaveable bowl versions.

Soups: A list of soups that are currently available in a canned and microwaveable bowl version are shown in **Appendix B** on page 118. These soup selections are perfect for the busy adult on the go. Soup selections are from three of the leading producers and therefore should be easy to find. Most have been taste-tested by the author and deemed acceptable to good.

Feel free to substitute other soup brands you favor in place of those indicated – provided the type of soup and calorie counts are similar to those specified in the *100-Day No-Cooking Diet*. For example, Day 68 calls for Campbell's Vegetable Soup (100 Calories), but if you prefer, you may substitute Amy's Chunky Vegetable Soup (120 Calories) – which is packaged in a not as convenient can. Notice in the previous example, the type of soup substituted was almost the same and the calorie count was off but close.

Healthy Foods: Since 1994 the FDA has allowed the term "healthy" to be placed on the labels of certain foods that are comparatively low in total and saturated fat, meet limits for sodium and cholesterol, and contain some other micronutrients. Note that many commercial soups are loaded with salt (sodium), the exceptions being Campbell's Healthy Request® soups, Healthy Choice soups and some canned Progresso lower sodium soups (not listed in this diet).

Warm Weather Substitutions: On warm and especially very hot days, you may want to substitute a sandwich, a tuna salad, or a salmon salad for the soup of the day.

Subway Sandwich: Recently, Subway sandwich shops have become quite common. Because some of the smaller 6" sandwich versions contain a reasonable number of calories. Three sandwiches are included in this diet: Black Forest Ham & Cheese (260 Calories), Roast Beef & Cheese (245 Calories), and Turkey Breast & Cheese (230 Calories).

Hot Pockets Wrap: Again these wraps contain a reasonable number or calories and you will find many in the lunch sections of this diet.

Dinner Guidelines

Most of the dinners in the *100-Day No-Cooking Diet* are centered on a frozen entrée from one of the three leading manufacturers (Healthy Choice, Lean Cuisine and Weight Watcher's Smart Ones) and therefore should be easily found in your local supermarket. Again most have been taste-tested by the author and judged acceptable to good.

As mentioned previously, a high percentage of the *100-Day No-Cooking Diet* is based on frozen entrees. Nearly 150 frozen entrees are listed in **Appendix D** page 122 at the end of this book.

About Bread: First understand that bread, more specifically whole-grain breads, are good sources of complex carbohydrates and dietary fiber, as well as several B vitamins (thiamin, riboflavin, niacin, and folate), vitamin E, and minerals (iron, magnesium and selenium). In recent years, however, sliced bread loaves have gotten larger, as have the bread slices inside these loaves. Just a few years ago the standard slice of bread contained about 70 Calories – now most are 100 plus Calories.

The *100-Day No-Cooking Diet* **requires whole-grain bread at 70 Calories per slice.** Quite a few bakers sell thin sliced or "light" sliced bread. The difficult part is finding a whole grain thin sliced or "light" bread (with about 70 Calories per slice). Whatever the brand, make sure the first word in the ingredient list is "whole." "Pepperidge Farm Small Slice 100% Whole Wheat" is a good choice. It's whole grain, has 70 Calories per slice and it tastes good too.

Have a Big-Bowl Salad

Yet another problem with nearly all frozen entrees is that they don't contain enough veggies. The solution is to have a "Big-Bowl Salad" at dinnertime with your frozen entrée. A typical "Big-Bowl Salad" is shown in the photo below.

To prepare a "Big-Bowl Salad" start with a relatively large soup bowl (with a volume of at least 24 ounces, or 3 cups). Add about 1½ cups of either green leaf lettuce, Romaine lettuce or a mesclun mix. Then add, as desired, veggies such as broccoli, celery, cucumber, onion, peppers, radish, spinach, tomato, or watercress, to make up the remaining 1½ cups, for a total of 3 cups. This vegetable combination will, on average, total about 100 Calories. You will be eating a "Big-Bowl Salad" every day at dinnertime. Remember that variety is the key to a nutritious diet. So be sure to vary the ingredients of the salad.

Top your "Big-Bowl Salad" with 2 tablespoons of any light salad dressing available at your local supermarket that contains no more than 25 Calories per tablespoon. Some of my favorite light salad dressings are:

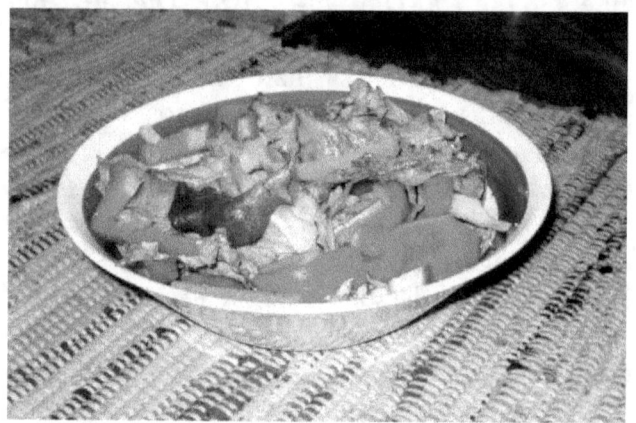

Big-Bowl Salad

- **Ken's Steakhouse Fat Free Raspberry Pecan**
- **Kraft Light Done Right House Italian**
- **Newman's Lighten Up! Balsamic Vinaigrette**
- **Wishbone Just 2 Good Honey Dijon**

Your "Big-Bowl Salad" with dressing will cost you roughly 150 Calories but will be packed with lots of health-giving vitamins, minerals and fiber.

Snack Guidelines

The *100-Day No-Cooking Diet* features a morning snack, an afternoon snack and an evening snack, every day. The main snacks are:

Non-fat Yogurt: Whatever brand you buy be sure to only eat 60 Calories of yogurt for your snack. (Shopping hint: Buy a large 32 oz container of non-fat yogurt, any flavor, and scoop out about 4 oz.)

Fresh Fruit in season: Choose an apple, pear, peach, plum, watermelon (1 cup), etc. You will be eating fruit just about every day. So vary the fruit that you select to get good array of micronutrients.

Handful of Unsalted Mixed Nuts: Nuts and seeds are loaded with protein and fiber. This book uses a "handful" as a convenient descriptor rather than something like "16 almonds = 100 Calories," but be aware that although nuts are a healthy food, nuts are also a high-calorie food. Buy mixed nuts in bulk to get a range of micronutrients. And please no salt. The last thing you need on this diet is more salt.

Skinny Cow Ice Cream Sandwich: This is a relatively low-calorie, low fat, yummy dairy-sweet snack.

Nature Valley Crunchy Granola bar: A sweet treat packed with whole grains, nuts and seeds. The bar contains about 90 Calories.

Popcorn Mini Bag: Popcorn is a tasty, nutritious high-fiber, filling snack. For a busy adult Orville Redenbacher's Smart Pop Popcorn Mini Bag and others are packaged in a convenient 110 Calorie portion you can just nuke and eat. But for the best popcorn we suggest you purchase a hot-air popper (about $25.00 at this writing) which will make a large batch of popcorn in a few minutes. For a snack, eat only 5 or 6 cups of the popcorn and store the rest for another day.

Your Night Out

Everyone deserves a break from the grind of preparing dinner after coming home from work. So the *100-Day No-Cooking Diet* gives you one night off per week! One night a week when you are encouraged to eat out. The diet is setup so that the night out usually occurs on Days 7, 14, 21, etc. Which day of the week you actually eat out depends on which day of the week you start the diet. So if you start the diet on a Monday, your night out will fall on a Sunday. If you would rather eat out on a work day, then start the diet on a Wednesday and your night off will be Tuesdays. Whatever night you eat out, however, some rules and caveats are in order – and these are covered in the next section.

Eating Out Caveats & Tips

You may eat out once a week. When you're on a diet, however, eating in a restaurant can be a challenge, in view of the fact that most restaurant portions are huge and can easily total more than 1,000 Calories. Because there are a limited number of frozen fish entrees available, if possible order fish on your night out. On the *100-Day No-Cooking Diet*, an eating-out calorie target will be specified. For example Day 7 of the 1,200 Calorie diet specifies a fish dinner and allows you 530 Calories – which can translate in a satisfying amount of food if you're careful. Here are some dinning-out strategies:

First order a broiled or baked fish dinner. Why? Because there are just not that many frozen-fish entrées sold in supermarkets and broiled or baked fish is generally lower in calories than a meat entrée. (If not fish order chicken.) And make sure you choose a restaurant where you have a fighting chance to achieve your calorie goal. Many restaurants have websites that post their menu. This allows you to select your meal before you get to the eatery. Once in a restaurant, with a waiter hovering nearby, you may not be able to quickly identify the healthiest options on the menu. But don't be rushed or intimidated by the waiter. Remember, it's his job to make sure you're happy with your meal. And even if you've researched your picks ahead of time, be clear about your preferences when you order. This way, if your order comes swimming in a creamy butter sauce, you won't feel guilty sending it back.

Some experienced dieters try to phone the restaurant ahead of time, at an off-hour like mid-afternoon, to see if they can pre-order a calorie-restricted meal. If you call, at a minimum, ask how various menu selections are prepared such as: "Is there butter, margarine, mayonnaise or cheese in the sauce? If so, can I have the sauce on the side?" and "Can veggies be steamed or cooked without fat?"

Most restaurant entrées are enormous. An alternative is to request a half-size or appetizer-size portion, or share a full-size entree with a dinning partner. And always order a simple straight-forward meal, such as broiled fish with steamed vegetables and brown rice. Tell the waiter you want no sauce, no gravy, nothing added. Then, knowing your calorie objective, and that most fish are about 50 Calories per ounce, most steamed vegetable servings average approximately 50 Calories per cup, and rice is about 100 Calories per ½ cup, decide how much to eat – and take the remainder home. If fresh fruit is not an option, decline dessert and have the evening snack (if any) specified in the meal plan for that day.

Incidentally, if you're on a budget and would rather not eat out just pick a frozen entrée from Appendix D; make a "Big-Bowl Salad," select a dessert from the Snacks Guidelines section.

Important Notes
1) Coffee or tea may be caffeinated or decaf. If desired, skim milk and a sugar substitute may be added to coffee or tea. And soy or almond milk may be used in place of cow's milk.

2) Fried eggs or scrambled eggs should be cooked in a pan coated with a non-stick cooking spray. Hard-boiled eggs may be substituted for fried, scrambled or soft-boiled eggs.

3) Cereals should be whole grain and unsweetened. At the top of the list are Old-fashioned Oatmeal, Wheatena and Shredded Wheat. Among other reasonably healthy choices are Cheerios, Wheat Chex, Wheaties, some Kashi cereals and Farina. When blueberries are in season, you may **substitute blueberries for raisins** added to your cereal. (Substitution ratio = 2 blueberries per raisin.)

4) Bread may be either plain or toasted whole grain, such as whole wheat, whole rye or pumpernickel. Look for whole grain varieties that contain 70 Calories per slice. If desired, bread may be sprayed with a zero-calorie butter substitute.

5) When soup is specified, have only one serving (8 ounces) unless otherwise noted. (Microwaveable bowls and cans usually contain about two servings.)

6) Use freely as desired: clear unsweetened coffee, clear unsweetened tea, water, seltzer water and any Diet soda or water, clear soups without fat, bouillon, and seasonings such as mustard, cinnamon, dill, herbs, red and black pepper, curry, vinegar, lemon juice and sections, and dill and sour pickles.

7) Use only lean cuts of meat trimmed of all visible fat. Poultry should be limited to chicken or turkey breasts (white meat only and skinless).

8) When canned tuna or salmon is specified, use only fish packed in water.

9) When the diet calls for turkey bacon, make sure the brand you buy has no more than 35 Calories per slice.

10) An unlimited amount of green salad may be eaten, but the salad dressing should be as specified.

11) If it's more convenient, any food item may be moved to any part of the day and combined with any meal or snack.

12) If you cannot find the exact item called for in the diet (because it's out of stock or discontinued), substitute a comparable food (of the same type and close caloric value).

13) Take a daily multi-vitamin/mineral supplement. This is important when you're on a diet – as a kind of insurance policy.

You Can Keep It Off

Within five years, more than 90 percent of all dieters regain every pound they have lost. Why? In most cases it's because after losing weight most people eventually revert to their pre-diet eating and exercising habits, and this inevitably leads to their regaining the weight they lost – and often more. The fact is the less you weigh, the less you need to eat to sustain your lower weight. A study, published in the Annals of Internal Medicine, that followed 4,000 people for three decades showed that in the long term, 80 percent of normal weight people eventually became overweight. The point being that you can never become complacent and must continually watch your weight. We are all at risk of becoming overweight.

As mentioned previously, the key to long-term weight control success is knowledge and understanding, combined of course with desire and self-discipline. Once more, for the full story see *Weight Control - U.S. Edition* by Vincent Antonetti, Ph.D., published by NoPaperPress.com. If you want to keep it off weight you have lost, or just maintain your weight, get a copy of the book *Weight Maintenance - U.S. Edition* by Vincent Antonetti, Ph.D., also by NoPaperPress.com, and absolutely the best weight maintenance book on the market.

1500-CALORIE DAILY MENUS

Day 1 1500 Calorie Meal Plan

BREAKFAST	Calories	Totals
Orange juice (½ cup)	50	
Wheaties (¾ cup) + ½ cup skim milk + ½ banana	190	
Whole-grain toast (1 slice) (See page 9)	70	
Coffee (See page 12)	10	320 Cal
SNACK		
Fresh fruit in season (apple, peach, etc)	70	
Coffee or tea	10	80 Cal
LUNCH		
Soup (Appendix B - page 118)	110	
String cheese (1 piece, any brand)*	80	
Whole-grain bread (1 slice)	70	
Coffee or tea	10	270 Cal
* Maximum of 80 Calories		
SNACK		
Handful unsalted mixed nuts	100	
Coffee or tea	10	110 Cal
DINNER		
Frozen Entrée (Appendix D - page 122)	290	
"Big-Bowl Salad" (Dressings - page 10)	150	
Whole grain bread (1 slice)	70	
Fresh fruit in season (apple, plum, etc)	70	
Water with lemon wedge	15	595 Cal
SNACK		
Popcorn Mini Bag**	110	
Coffee or tea	10	120 Cal
** Such as Orville Redenbacher's Smart Pop.		1495 Cal

Day 2 1500 Calorie Meal Plan		
BREAKFAST	Calories	Totals
Fresh or frozen strawberries (½ cup)	25	
Kashi Go Lean Waffles* (2)	150	
Morningstar Breakfast Sausage Link*	80	
Light Syrup (2 Tbsp)	50	
Coffee	10	315 Cal
SNACK		
Yogurt (4 oz, non-fat, any flavor - **see page 10**)	60	
Coffee or tea	10	70 Cal
LUNCH		
Ham (2 oz) with mustard on 2 slices rye bread	300	
Laughing Cow Light Cheese* (1 wedge)	35	
Fresh fruit in season (pear, peach, etc)	70	
Coffee or tea	10	415 Cal
SNACK		
Handful unsalted mixed nuts	100	
Coffee or tea	10	110 Cal
DINNER		
Frozen Entrée (Appendix D **- page 122**)	200	
"Big-Bowl Salad"	150	
Whole-grain bread (1 slice)	70	
Water	0	440 Cal
SNACK		
Skinny Cow Ice Cream Sandwich*	160	
Coffee or tea	10	170 Cal
* If unavailable an equivalent dessert.		1500 Cal

Day 3 1500 Calorie Meal Plan		
BREAKFAST	Calories	Totals
Grapefruit (½)	75	
Scrambled egg (**See page 13**)	80	
Turkey bacon - 1 slice (**See page 13**)	35	
Whole-grain toast (1 slice)	70	
Coffee	10	270 Cal
SNACK		
Yogurt (4 oz, non-fat, any flavor)	60	
Coffee or tea	10	70 Cal
LUNCH		
Salad (3 oz canned tuna, 1 tsp Evoo, onions, celery)	175	
Rye bread (1 slice)	70	
Laughing Cow Light Cheese* (1 wedge)	35	
Hot or iced tea	10	290 Cal
SNACK		
Handful unsalted mixed nuts	100	
Coffee or tea	10	110 Cal
DINNER		
Frozen Entrée (Appendix D - **page 122**)	260	
"Big-Bowl Salad"	150	
Whole-grain bread (1 slice)	70	
Fresh fruit in season (apple, peach, etc)	70	
Water with lemon wedge	15	565 Cal
SNACK		
Kashi TLC Crunchy Granola Bar*	180	
Coffee or tea	10	190 Cal
* If unavailable an equivalent dessert.		1495 Cal

Day 4 1500 Calorie Meal Plan		
BREAKFAST	Calories	Totals
Grapefruit (½)	75	
Cheerios (1 cup) + ½ cup skim milk + about 15 raisins*	190	
Coffee	10	275 Cal
SNACK		
Handful unsalted mixed nuts	100	
Coffee or tea	10	110 Cal
LUNCH		
Cottage cheese (1 cup low fat)	180	
Fresh fruit in season (apple, peach, etc)	70	
Small whole-grain roll	80	
Coffee or tea	10	340 Cal
SNACK		
Kashi TLC Crunchy Granola Bar**	180	
Coffee or tea	10	190 Cal
** If unavailable substitute an equivalent dessert.		
DINNER		
Frozen Entrée (Appendix D - **page 122**)	270	
"Big-Bowl Salad"	150	
Whole-grain bread (1 slice)	70	
Water with lemon wedge	15	505 Cal
SNACK		
Fresh fruit in season (apple, plum, etc)	70	
Coffee or tea	10	80 Cal
* See Notes page 13 re substituting blueberries for raisins.		1500 Cal

Day 5 1500 Calorie Meal Plan		
BREAKFAST	Calories	Totals
Cantaloupe (½ medium)	50	
Fried egg (2 eggs)	160	
Toasted raisin bread (1 slice)	75	
Coffee	10	295 Cal
SNACK		
Yogurt (4 oz, non-fat, any flavor)	60	
Coffee or tea	10	70 Cal
LUNCH		
Subway 6" (Ham, Cheese + veggies)*	260	
Banana (1 medium)	100	
Water	0	360 Cal
* Half of 9-grain roll.		
SNACK		
Fresh fruit in season (apple, plum, etc)	70	
Coffee or tea	10	80 Cal
DINNER		
Frozen Entrée (Appendix D - **page 122**)	210	
"Big-Bowl Salad"	150	
Small whole-grain roll	80	
Glass of wine (4 oz)	100	
Water	0	540 Cal
SNACK		
Skinny Cow Ice Cream Sandwich**	160	
Coffee or tea	10	170 Cal
** If unavailable an equivalent dessert.		1515 Cal

Day 6 1500 Calorie Meal Plan

BREAKFAST	Calories	Totals
Tomato juice (½ cup)	20	
Shredded Wheat (1 cup) + ½ cup skim milk + ½ banana	265	
Coffee	10	295 Cal
SNACK		
Yogurt (4 oz, non-fat, any flavor)	60	
Coffee or tea	10	70 Cal
LUNCH		
Chorizo, Egg & Cheese*	260	
Fresh fruit in season (apple, peach, plum, etc)	70	
Diet soda or water	0	330 Cal
* Hot Pockets (wrap). If unavailable an equivalent food.		
SNACK		
Handful unsalted mixed nuts	100	
Coffee or tea	10	110 Cal
DINNER		
Frozen Entrée (Appendix D **- page 122**)	260	
"Big-Bowl Salad"	150	
Whole-grain bread (1 slice)	70	
Fresh blueberries, cherries or grapes (1 cup)	100	
Water with lemon wedge	15	595 Cal
SNACK		
Nature Valley Crunchy Granola Bar**	95	
Coffee or tea	10	105 Cal
** One bar only. If unavailable an equivalent dessert.		1505 Cal

Day 7 1500 Calorie Meal Plan		
BREAKFAST	Calories	Totals
Cantaloupe (½ medium)	50	
Oatmeal (**½ cup dry**) + **½ cup skim milk** + **about 15**	220	
Coffee	10	280 Cal
SNACK		
Fresh fruit in season (peach, plum, etc)	70	
Coffee or tea	10	80 Cal
LUNCH		
Frozen Entrée (Appendix D **- page 122**)	330	
Water with lemon wedge	15	345 Cal
SNACK		
Coffee or tea	10	10 Cal
DINNER		
Eat Out – Fish dinner (**See page 11**)		
– Maximum allowable calories	670	670 Cal
SNACK		
100 Calorie Pack Cookies*	100	
Coffee or tea	10	110 Cal
* Such as Nabisco Oreos, Chips Ahoy, etc		1495 Cal

Day 8 1500 Calorie Meal Plan

BREAKFAST	Calories	Totals
Orange juice (½ cup)	50	
Wheat Chex (¾ cup) + ½ cup skim milk + ½ banana	250	
Coffee	10	310 Cal
SNACK		
Fresh fruit in season (peach, plum, etc)	70	
Coffee or tea	10	80 Cal
LUNCH		
Soup (Appendix B - **page 118**)	120	
String cheese (1 piece, any brand)	80	
Whole-grain bread (1 slice)	70	
Coffee or tea	10	280 Cal
SNACK		
Handful unsalted mixed nuts	100	
Coffee or tea	10	110 Cal
DINNER		
Frozen Entrée (Appendix D - **page 122**)	300	
"Big-Bowl Salad"	150	
Whole-grain bread (1 slice)	70	
Fresh fruit in season (apple, plum, etc)	70	
Water with lemon wedge	15	605 Cal
SNACK		
Popcorn Mini Bag*	110	
Coffee or tea	10	120 Cal
* Such as Orville Redenbacher's Smart Pop.		1505 Cal

Day 9 1500 Calorie Meal Plan		
BREAKFAST	Calories	Totals
Orange juice (½ cup)	50	
Kashi Go Lean Waffles (2)	150	
Morningstar Breakfast Sausage Link	80	
Light Syrup (2 Tbsp)	50	
Coffee	10	340 Cal
SNACK		
Yogurt (4 oz, non-fat, any flavor)	60	
Coffee or tea	10	70 Cal
LUNCH		
Chicken, Bacon Ranch*	270	
Fresh fruit in season (apple, peach, plum, etc)	70	
Diet soda or water	0	340 Cal
* Hot Pockets (wrap). If unavailable an equivalent food.		
SNACK		
Handful unsalted mixed nuts	100	
Coffee or tea	10	110 Cal
DINNER		
Frozen Entrée (Appendix D - **page 122**)	250	
"Big-Bowl Salad"	150	
Whole-grain bread (1 slice)	70	
Water with lemon wedge	15	485 Cal
SNACK		
Skinny Cow Ice Cream Sandwich**	160	
Coffee or tea	10	170 Cal
** If unavailable an equivalent dessert.		1515 Cal

Day 10 1500 Calorie Meal Plan

BREAKFAST	Calories	Totals
Grapefruit (½)	75	
Soft-boiled egg	80	
Whole-grain toast (1 slice)	70	
Coffee	10	235 Cal
SNACK		
Yogurt (4 oz, non-fat, any flavor)	60	
Coffee or tea	10	70 Cal
LUNCH		
Subway 6" (Roast Beef, Cheese + veggies)*	245	
Fresh fruit in season (apple, plum, etc)	70	
Water with lemon wedge	15	330 Cal
* Half of 9-grain roll.		
SNACK		
Handful unsalted mixed nuts	100	
Coffee or tea	10	110 Cal
DINNER		
Frozen Entrée (Appendix D - **page 122**)	290	
"Big-Bowl Salad"	150	
Whole-grain bread (1 slice)	70	
Fresh fruit in season (apple, peach, etc)	70	
Water with lemon wedge	15	595 Cal
SNACK		
Kashi TLC Chewy Granola Bar**	140	
Coffee or tea	10	150 Cal
** If unavailable an equivalent dessert.		1490 Cal

Day 11 1500 Calorie Meal Plan

BREAKFAST	Calories	Totals
Fresh sliced orange	75	
Cheerios (1 cup) + ½ cup skim milk + about 15 raisins	190	
Whole grain toast (1 slice)	70	
Coffee	10	345 Cal
SNACK		
Handful unsalted mixed nuts	100	
Coffee or tea	10	110 Cal
LUNCH		
Cottage cheese (1 cup low fat)	180	
Fresh fruit in season (apple, plum, etc)	70	
Small whole-grain roll	80	
Water	10	330 Cal
SNACK		
Kashi TLC Chewy Granola Bar	140	
Coffee or tea	10	150 Cal
DINNER		
Frozen Entrée (Appendix D - **page 122**)	220	
"Big-Bowl Salad"	150	
Whole-grain bread (1 slice)	70	
Water	0	440 Cal
SNACK		
Popcorn Mini Bag	110	
Coffee or tea	10	120 Cal
		1505 Cal

Day 12 1500 Calorie Meal Plan

BREAKFAST	Calories	Totals
Grapefruit (½)	75	
Scrambled egg	80	
Turkey bacon (1 slice)	35	
Whole-grain toast (1 slice)	70	
Coffee	10	270 Cal
SNACK		
Fresh fruit in season (peach, plum, etc)	70	
Coffee or tea	10	80 Cal
LUNCH		
Salad (3 oz canned tuna, 1 tsp Evoo, onions, celery)	175	
Rye bread (1 slice)	70	
Banana (medium)	100	
Diet soda or water	0	345 Cal
SNACK		
Yogurt (4 oz, non-fat, any flavor)	60	
Coffee or tea	10	70 Cal
DINNER		
Frozen Entrée (Appendix D - **page 122**)	350	
"Big-Bowl Salad"	150	
Fresh fruit in season (apple, plum, etc)	70	
Water	0	570 Cal
SNACK		
Skinny Cow Ice Cream Sandwich	160	
Coffee or tea	10	170 Cal
		1505 Cal

Day 13 1500 Calorie Meal Plan

BREAKFAST	Calories	Totals
Orange juice (½ cup)	50	
Shredded Wheat **(1 cup)** + ½ cup skim milk + **½ banana**	260	
Coffee	10	320 Cal
SNACK		
Fresh fruit in season (pear, plum, etc)	70	
Coffee or tea	10	80 Cal
LUNCH		
Peanut butter (2 Tbsp) on 2 slices bread	340	
Skim milk (4 oz)	45	385 Cal
SNACK		
Kashi TLC Chewy Granola Bar	140	
Coffee or tea	10	150 Cal
DINNER		
Frozen Entrée (Appendix D **- page 122**)	190	
"Big-Bowl Salad"	150	
Whole-grain bread (1 slice)	70	
Water with lemon wedge	15	425 Cal
SNACK		
Graham crackers (4 squares)	120	
Coffee or tea	10	130 Cal
		1490 Cal

Day 14 1500 Calorie Meal Plan		
BREAKFAST	Calories	Totals
Cantaloupe (½ medium)	50	
Oatmeal (½ cup dry) + ½ cup skim milk + 15 raisins*	220	
Coffee	10	280 Cal
SNACK		
Fresh fruit in season (apple, peach, etc)	70	
Coffee or tea	10	80 Cal
LUNCH		
Frozen Entrée (Appendix D - **page 122**)	330	
Diet soda or water	0	330 Cal
SNACK		
Yogurt (4 oz, non-fat, any flavor)	60	
Coffee or tea	10	70 Cal
DINNER		
Eat Out – Fish dinner (**See page 11**)		
– Maximum allowable calories	620	620 Cal
SNACK		
100-Calorie Pack Cookies*	100	
Coffee or tea	10	110 Cal
* **For example, Nabisco Oreo/Chips Ahoy, etc**		1500 Cal

Day 15 1500 Calorie Meal Plan

BREAKFAST	Calories	Totals
Fresh sliced orange	75	
Wheaties (¾ cup) + ½ cup skim milk + ½ banana	190	
Whole-grain toast (1 slice)	70	
Coffee	10	345 Cal
SNACK		
Fresh fruit in season (apple, plum, etc)	70	
Coffee or tea	10	80 Cal
LUNCH		
Soup (Appendix B **- page 118**)	130	
String cheese (1 piece, any brand)*	80	
Small whole-grain roll	80	
Coffee or tea	10	300 Cal
* Maximum of 80 Calories.		
SNACK		
Handful unsalted mixed nuts	100	
Coffee or tea	10	110 Cal
DINNER		
Frozen Entrée (Appendix D **- page 122**)	330	
"Big-Bowl Salad"	150	
Fresh fruit in season (peach, plum, etc)	70	
Water	0	550 Cal
SNACK		
Pop Popcorn Mini Bag	110	
Coffee or tea	10	120 Cal
		1505 Cal

Day 16 1500 Calorie Meal Plan		
BREAKFAST	Calories	Totals
Orange juice (½ cup)	50	
Wheat Chex (¾ cup) + ½ cup skim milk + ½ banana	250	
Coffee	10	310 Cal
SNACK		
Yogurt (4 oz, non-fat, any flavor)	60	
Coffee or tea	10	70 Cal
LUNCH		
Ham & Cheddar*	270	
Fresh fruit in season (apple, plum, etc)	70	
Coffee or tea	10	350 Cal
* Hot Pockets (wrap)		
SNACK		
Handful unsalted mixed nuts	100	
Coffee or tea	10	110 Cal
DINNER		
Frozen Entrée (Appendix D **- page 122**)	240	
"Big-Bowl Salad"	150	
Whole-grain bread (1 slice)	70	
Fresh fruit in season (apple, pear, etc)	70	
Water with lemon wedge	15	545 Cal
SNACK		
Skinny Cow Fudge Ice Cream Bar**	110	
Coffee or tea	10	120 Cal
** If unavailable an equivalent dessert.		1505 Cal

Day 17 1500 Calorie Meal Plan

BREAKFAST	Calories	Totals
Cantaloupe (½ medium)	50	
Scrambled egg	80	
Turkey bacon (2 slices)	70	
Toasted raisin bread (1 slice)	75	
Coffee	10	285 Cal
SNACK		
Yogurt (4 oz, non-fat, any flavor)	60	
Coffee or tea	10	70 Cal
LUNCH		
Soup (Appendix B - **page 118**)	170	
String cheese (1 piece, any brand)	80	
Nature Valley Crunchy Granola bar	95	
Coffee or tea	10	355 Cal
SNACK		
Handful unsalted mixed nuts	100	
Coffee or tea	10	110 Cal
DINNER		
Frozen Entrée (Appendix D - **page 122**)	270	
"Big-Bowl Salad"	150	
Whole-grain bread (1 slice)	70	
Fresh fruit in season (apple, plum, etc)	70	
Coffee or tea	10	570 Cal
SNACK		
Popcorn Mini Bag	110	
Coffee or tea	10	120 Cal
		1510 Cal

Day 18 1500 Calorie Meal Plan		
BREAKFAST	Calories	Totals
Grapefruit (½)	75	
Cheerios (1 cup) + ½ cup skim milk + about 15 raisins	190	
Coffee	10	275 Cal
SNACK		
Handful unsalted mixed nuts	100	
Coffee or tea	10	110 Cal
LUNCH		
Cottage cheese (1 cup low fat)	180	
Fresh fruit in season (apple, plum, etc)	70	
Small whole-grain roll	80	
Diet soda or water	0	330 Cal
SNACK		
Kashi TLC Chewy Granola Bar	140	
Coffee or tea	10	150 Cal
DINNER		
Frozen Entrée (Appendix D - **page 122**)	210	
"Big-Bowl Salad"	150	
Whole-grain bread (1 slice)	70	
Fresh fruit in season (peach, plum, etc)	70	
Water with lemon wedge	15	515 Cal
SNACK		
Popcorn Mini Bag	110	
Coffee or tea	10	120 Cal
		1500 Cal

Day 19 1500 Calorie Meal Plan

BREAKFAST	Calories	Totals
Grapefruit (½)	75	
Fried egg	80	
Whole grain toast (2 slices)	140	
Coffee	10	305 Cal
SNACK		
Yogurt (4 oz, non-fat, any flavor)	60	
Coffee or tea	10	70 Cal
LUNCH		
Subway 6" (Roast Beef, Cheese + veggies)*	245	
Fresh fruit in season (apple, pear, etc)	70	
Diet soda (or water)	0	315 Cal
* Half of 9-grain roll.		
SNACK		
Handful unsalted mixed nuts	100	
Coffee or tea	10	110 Cal
DINNER		
Frozen Entrée (Appendix D - **page 122**)	290	
"Big-Bowl Salad"	150	
Fresh fruit in season (peach, plum, etc)	70	
Water with lemon wedge	15	525 Cal
SNACK		
Skinny Cow Ice Cream Sandwich	160	
Coffee or tea	10	170 Cal
		1495 Cal

Day 20 1500 Calorie Meal Plan		
BREAKFAST	Calories	Totals
Tomato juice (½ cup)	20	
Shredded Wheat (**1 cup**) + ½ cup skim milk + ½ banana	260	
Coffee	10	290 Cal
SNACK		
Yogurt (4 oz, non-fat, any flavor)	60	
Coffee or tea	10	70 Cal
LUNCH		
Chorizo, Egg & Cheese*	260	
Fresh fruit in season (pear, plum, etc)	70	
Diet soda (or water)	0	330 Cal
* Hot Pockets (wrap)		
SNACK		
Handful unsalted mixed nuts	100	
Coffee or tea	10	110 Cal
DINNER		
Frozen Entrée (Appendix D - **page 122**)	270	
"Big-Bowl Salad"	150	
Whole-grain bread (1 slice)	70	
Fresh fruit in season (apple, peach, etc)	70	
Water	0	560 Cal
SNACK		
Kashi TLC Chewy Granola Bar	140	140 Cal
		1500 Cal

Day 21 1500 Calorie Meal Plan

BREAKFAST	Calories	Totals
Cantaloupe (½ medium)	50	
Oatmeal (**½ cup dry**) + **½ cup skim milk** + **15 raisins**	220	
Coffee	10	280 Cal
SNACK		
Fresh fruit in season (pear, plum, etc)	70	
Coffee or tea	10	80 Cal
LUNCH		
Frozen Entrée (Appendix D **- page 122**)	290	
Diet soda or water	0	290 Cal
SNACK		
Yogurt (4 oz, non-fat, any flavor)	60	
Coffee or tea	10	70 Cal
DINNER		
Eat Out – Fish dinner (**See page 11**)		
– Maximum allowable calories	670	670 Cal
SNACK		
100-Calorie Pack Cookies	100	
Coffee or tea	10	110 Cal
		1500 Cal

Day 22 1500 Calorie Meal Plan		
BREAKFAST	Calories	Totals
Cantaloupe (½ medium)	50	
Wheat Chex (¾ cup) + ½ cup skim milk + ½ banana	250	
Coffee	10	310 Cal
SNACK		
Fresh fruit in season (peach, plum, etc)	70	
Coffee or tea	10	80 Cal
LUNCH		
Salad (3 oz canned tuna, 1 tsp Evoo, onions, celery)	175	
String cheese (1 piece, any brand - 80 Cal max)	80	
Rye bread (1 slice)	70	
Diet soda or water	0	325 Cal
SNACK		
Handful unsalted mixed nuts	100	
Coffee or tea	10	110 Cal
DINNER		
Frozen Entrée (Appendix D - **page 122**)	260	
"Big-Bowl Salad"	150	
Whole-grain bread (1 slice)	70	
Fresh fruit in season (apple, pear, etc)	70	
Water with lemon wedge	15	565 Cal
SNACK		
Popcorn Mini Bag	110	
Coffee or tea	10	120 Cal
		1510 Cal

Day 23 1500 Calorie Meal Plan

BREAKFAST	Calories	Totals
Fresh or frozen strawberries (½ cup)	25	
Kashi Go Lean Waffles (2)	150	
Morningstar Breakfast Sausage Link	80	
Light Syrup (2 Tbsp)	50	
Coffee	10	315 Cal
SNACK		
Yogurt (4 oz, non-fat, any flavor)	60	
Coffee or tea	10	70 Cal
LUNCH		
Ham (2 oz) with mustard on 2 slices rye bread	300	
Pickle spear	0	
Fresh fruit in season (peach, plum, etc)	70	
Hot or iced tea	10	380 Cal
SNACK		
Handful unsalted mixed nuts	100	
Coffee or tea	10	110 Cal
DINNER		
Frozen Entrée (Appendix D - **page 122**)	250	
"Big-Bowl Salad"	150	
Fresh fruit in season (peach, plum, etc)	70	
Water	0	470 Cal
SNACK		
Skinny Cow Ice Cream Sandwich	160	
Coffee or tea	10	170 Cal
		1515 Cal

Day 24 1500 Calorie Meal Plan		
BREAKFAST	Calories	Totals
Orange juice (½ cup)	50	
Soft-boiled egg	80	
Whole-grain toast (1 slice)	70	
Coffee	10	210 Cal
SNACK		
Fresh fruit in season (apple, plum, etc)	70	
Coffee or tea	10	80 Cal
LUNCH		
Soup (Appendix B - **page 118**)*	260	
String cheese (1 piece, any brand)	80	
Small whole-grain roll	80	
Coffee or tea	10	430 Cal
* Enjoy 2 servings of 130 Cal soup.		
SNACK		
Yogurt (4 oz, non-fat, any flavor)	60	
Coffee or tea	10	70 Cal
DINNER		
Frozen Entrée (Appendix D - **page 122**)	260	
"Big-Bowl Salad"	150	
Whole-grain bread (1 slice)	70	
Fresh fruit in season (pear, plum, etc)	70	
Water	0	550 Cal
SNACK		
Skinny Cow Ice Cream Sandwich	160	
Coffee or tea	10	170 Cal
		1510 Cal

Day 25 1500 Calorie Meal Plan

BREAKFAST	Calories	Totals
Grapefruit (½)	75	
Cheerios (1 cup) + ½ cup skim milk + about 15 raisins	190	
Coffee	10	275 Cal
SNACK		
Handful unsalted mixed nuts	100	
Coffee or tea	10	110 Cal
LUNCH		
Cottage cheese (1 cup low fat)	180	
Fresh fruit in season (apple, plum, etc)	70	
Whole-grain bread (1 slice)	70	
Coffee or tea	10	330 Cal
SNACK		
Kashi TLC Chewy Granola Bar	140	
Coffee or tea	10	150 Cal
DINNER		
Frozen Entrée (Appendix D **- page 122**)	280	
"Big-Bowl Salad"	150	
Small whole-grain roll	80	
Water	0	510 Cal
SNACK		
Popcorn Mini Bag	110	
Coffee or tea	10	120 Cal
		1495 Cal

Day 26 1500 Calorie Meal Plan

BREAKFAST	Calories	Totals
Cantaloupe (½ medium)	50	
Scrambled egg	80	
Toasted whole-grain bread (1 slice)	70	
Coffee	10	210 Cal
SNACK		
Yogurt (4 oz, non-fat, any flavor)	60	
Coffee or tea	10	70 Cal
LUNCH		
Subway 6" (Ham, Cheese + veggies)	260	
Fresh fruit in season (apple, peach, etc)	70	
Water with lemon wedge	15	345 Cal
* Half of 9-grain roll.		
SNACK		
Handful unsalted mixed nuts	100	
Coffee or tea	10	110 Cal
DINNER		
Frozen Entrée (Appendix D **- page 122**)	310	
"Big-Bowl Salad"	150	
Whole-grain bread (1 slice)	70	
Fresh fruit in season (apple, peach, plum, etc)	70	
Water	0	600 Cal
SNACK		
Skinny Cow Ice Cream Sandwich	160	
Coffee or tea	10	170 Cal
		1505 Cal

Day 27 1500 Calorie Meal Plan

BREAKFAST	Calories	Totals
Cantaloupe (½ medium)	50	
Oatmeal (**½ cup dry**) + **½ cup skim milk** + **15 raisins**	220	
Coffee	10	280 Cal
SNACK		
Yogurt (4 oz, non-fat, any flavor)	60	
Coffee or tea	10	70 Cal
LUNCH		
Chicken Broccoli & Cheese*	270	
Fresh fruit in season (pear, plum, etc)	70	
Diet soda or water	10	330 Cal
* **Hot Pockets (wrap).**		
SNACK		
Handful unsalted mixed nuts	100	
Coffee or tea	10	110 Cal
DINNER		
Frozen Entrée (Appendix D - **page 122**)	260	
"Big-Bowl Salad"	150	
Whole-grain bread (1 slice)	70	
Fresh fruit in season (apple, peach, etc)	70	
Water with lemon wedge	15	565 Cal
SNACK		
Kashi TLC Chewy Granola Bar	140	
Coffee or tea	10	150 Cal
		1505 Cal

Day 28 1500 Calorie Meal Plan		
BREAKFAST	Calories	Totals
Tomato juice (½ cup)	20	
Shredded Wheat **(1 cup)** + **½ cup skim milk** + **½ banana**	260	
Coffee	10	290 Cal
SNACK		
Fresh fruit in season (apple, plum, etc)	70	
Coffee or tea	10	80 Cal
LUNCH		
Frozen Entrée (Appendix D **- page 122**)	280	
Diet soda or water	0	280 Cal
SNACK		
Yogurt (4 oz, non-fat, any flavor)	60	
Coffee or tea	10	70 Cal
DINNER		
Eat Out – Fish dinner **(See page 11)**		
– Maximum allowable calories	670	670 Cal
SNACK		
100-Calorie Pack Cookies	100	
Coffee or tea	10	110 Cal
		1500 Cal

Day 29 1500 Calorie Meal Plan		
BREAKFAST	Calories	Totals
Orange juice (½ cup)	50	
Wheaties (¾ cup) + ½ cup skim milk + ½ banana	190	
Whole-grain toast (1 slice)	70	
Coffee	10	320 Cal
SNACK		
Fresh fruit in season (peach, plum, etc)	70	
Coffee or tea	10	80 Cal
LUNCH		
Salad (3 oz canned tuna, 1 tsp Evoo, onions, celery)	175	
String cheese (1 piece, any brand - 80 Cal max)	80	
Rye bread (1 slice)	70	
Diet soda or water	0	325 Cal
SNACK		
Handful unsalted mixed nuts	100	
Coffee or tea	10	110 Cal
DINNER		
Frozen Entrée (Appendix D - **page 122**)	240	
"Big-Bowl Salad"	150	
Whole-grain bread (1 slice)	70	
Fresh fruit in season (apple, peach. etc)	70	
Water with lemon wedge	15	545 Cal
SNACK		
Popcorn Mini Bag	110	
Coffee or tea	10	120 Cal
		1500 Cal

Day 30 1500 Calorie Meal Plan

BREAKFAST	Calories	Totals
Orange juice (½ cup)	50	
Kashi Go Lean Waffles (2)	150	
Morningstar Breakfast Sausage Link	80	
Light Syrup (2 Tbsp)	50	
Coffee	10	340 Cal
SNACK		
Yogurt (4 oz, non-fat, any flavor)	60	
Coffee or tea	10	70 Cal
LUNCH		
Chicken, Bacon Ranch*	270	
Fresh fruit in season (apple, plum, etc)	70	
Diet soda (or water)	0	340 Cal
* Hot Pockets (wrap).		
SNACK		
Handful unsalted mixed nuts	100	
Coffee or tea	10	110 Cal
DINNER		
Frozen Entrée (Appendix D - **page 122**)	180	
"Big-Bowl Salad"	150	
Whole-grain bread (1 slice)	70	
Fresh fruit in season (peach, pear, etc)	70	
Water	0	490Cal
SNACK		
Skinny Cow Ice Cream Sandwich	160	
Coffee or tea	10	170 Cal
		1500 Cal

Day 31 1500 Calorie Meal Plan

BREAKFAST	Calories	Totals
Orange juice (½ cup)	50	
Cheerios (1 cup) + ½ cup skim milk + about 15 raisins	190	
Whole-grain toast (1 slice)	70	
Coffee	10	320 Cal
SNACK		
Fresh fruit in season (peach, plum, etc)	70	
Coffee or tea	10	80 Cal
LUNCH		
Soup (Appendix B - page 118)	100	
String cheese (1 piece, any brand)	80	
Whole-grain bread (1 slice)	70	
Coffee or tea	10	260 Cal
SNACK		
Handful unsalted mixed nuts	100	
Coffee or tea	10	110 Cal
DINNER		
Frozen Entrée (Appendix D - page 122)	310	
"Big-Bowl Salad"	150	
Whole grain bread (1 slice)	70	
Fresh fruit in season (apple, peach, etc)	70	
Water	0	600 Cal
SNACK		
Popcorn Mini Bag	110	
Coffee or tea	10	120 Cal
		1490 Cal

Day 32 1500 Calorie Meal Plan

BREAKFAST	Calories	Totals
Orange juice (½ cup)	50	
Kashi Go Lean Waffles (2)	150	
Morningstar Breakfast Sausage Link	80	
Light Syrup (2 Tbsp)	50	
Coffee	10	340 Cal
SNACK		
Yogurt (4 oz, non-fat, any flavor)	60	
Coffee or tea	10	70 Cal
LUNCH		
Ham (2 oz) with mustard on 2 slices rye bread	300	
Laughing Cow Light Cheese (1 wedge)	35	
Fresh fruit in season (apple, pear, etc)	70	
Hot or iced tea	10	415 Cal
SNACK		
Handful unsalted mixed nuts	100	
Coffee or tea	10	110 Cal
DINNER		
Frozen Entrée (Appendix D - **page 122**)	180	
"Big-Bowl Salad"	150	
Whole grain bread (1 slice)	70	
Water	0	400 Cal
SNACK		
Skinny Cow Ice Cream Sandwich	160	
Coffee or tea	10	170 Cal
		1505 Cal

Day 33 1500 Calorie Meal Plan

BREAKFAST	Calories	Totals
Grapefruit (½)	75	
Fried egg	80	
Turkey bacon (1 slice)	35	
Whole-grain toast (1 slice)	70	
Coffee	10	270 Cal
SNACK		
Yogurt (4 oz, non-fat, any flavor)	60	
Coffee or tea	10	70 Cal
LUNCH		
Salad (3 oz canned tuna, 1 tsp Evoo, onions, celery)	175	
Rye bread (1 slice)	70	
Small bunch of grapes	65	
Coffee or tea	10	320 Cal
SNACK		
Handful unsalted mixed nuts	100	
Coffee or tea	10	110 Cal
DINNER		
Frozen Entrée (Appendix D - **page 122**)	260	
"Big-Bowl Salad"	150	
Whole-grain bread (1 slice)	70	
Fresh fruit in season (apple, peach, etc)	70	
Water	0	550 Cal
SNACK		
Kashi TLC Crunchy Granola Bar	180	
Coffee or tea	10	190 Cal
		1510 Cal

Day 34 1500 Calorie Meal Plan		
BREAKFAST	Calories	Totals
Grapefruit (½)	75	
Wheaties (¾ cup) + ½ cup skim milk + ½ banana	190	
Coffee	10	275 Cal
SNACK		
Kashi TLC Crunchy Granola Bar	180	
Coffee or tea	10	190 Cal
LUNCH		
Subway 6" (Ham, Cheese + veggies)*	260	
Fresh fruit in season (apple, plum, etc)	70	
Coffee or tea	10	340 Cal
SNACK		
Handful unsalted mixed nuts	100	
Coffee or tea	10	110 Cal
DINNER		
Frozen Entrée (Appendix D - **page 122**)	270	
"Big-Bowl Salad"	150	
Whole-grain bread (1 slice)	70	
Water with lemon wedge	15	500 Cal
SNACK		
Fresh fruit in season (pear, plum, etc)	70	
Coffee or tea	10	80 Cal
		1495 Cal

Day 35 1500 Calorie Meal Plan

BREAKFAST	Calories	Totals
Cantaloupe (½ medium)	50	
Scrambled egg	80	
Toasted raisin bread (1 slice)	75	
Coffee	10	215 Cal
SNACK		
Yogurt (4 oz, non-fat, any flavor)	60	
Coffee or tea	10	70 Cal
LUNCH		
Soup (Appendix B **- page 118**)	280	
Whole-grain bread (1 slice)	70	
Banana (1 medium)	100	
Water	0	450 Cal
* Enjoy 2 servings of 140 Cal soup.		
SNACK		
Fresh fruit in season (peach, pear, etc)	70	
Coffee or tea	10	80 Cal
DINNER		
Frozen Entrée (Appendix D **- page 122**)	190	
"Big-Bowl Salad"	150	
Small whole-grain roll	80	
Glass of wine (4 oz)	100	
Water	0	520 Cal
SNACK		
Skinny Cow Ice Cream Sandwich	160	
Coffee or tea	10	170 Cal
		1505 Cal

Day 36 1500 Calorie Meal Plan

BREAKFAST	Calories	Totals
Tomato juice (½ cup)	20	
Shredded Wheat **(1 cup) + ½ cup skim milk + ½ banana**	265	
Coffee	10	295 Cal
SNACK		
Yogurt (4 oz, non-fat, any flavor)	60	
Coffee or tea	10	70 Cal
LUNCH		
Chicken Pot Pie*	230	
Fresh fruit in season (apple, peach, etc)	70	
Hot or iced tea	10	310 Cal
* Hot Pockets (wrap)		
SNACK		
Handful unsalted mixed nuts	100	
Coffee or tea	10	110 Cal
DINNER		
Frozen Entrée (Appendix D **- page 122**)	270	
"Big-Bowl Salad"	150	
Whole-grain bread (1 slice)	70	
Fresh blueberries, cherries or grapes (1 cup)	100	
Water with lemon wedge	15	605 Cal
SNACK		
Nature Valley Crunchy Granola bar	95	
Coffee or tea	10	105 Cal
		1495 Cal

Day 37 1500 Calorie Meal Plan

BREAKFAST	Calories	Totals
Cantaloupe (½ medium)	50	
Oatmeal (**½ cup dry**) + **½ cup skim milk** + **15 raisins**	220	
Coffee	10	280 Cal
SNACK		
Fresh fruit in season (apple, plum, etc)	70	
Coffee or tea	10	80 Cal
LUNCH		
Frozen Entrée (Appendix D **- page 122**)	290	
Diet soda or water	0	290 Cal
SNACK		
Yogurt (4 oz, non-fat, any flavor)	60	
Coffee or tea	10	70 Cal
DINNER		
Eat Out – Fish dinner (**See page 11**)		
– Maximum allowable calories	670	670 Cal
SNACK		
100-Calorie Pack Cookies	100	
Coffee or tea	10	110 Cal
		1500 Cal

Day 38 1500 Calorie Meal Plan

BREAKFAST	Calories	Totals
Orange juice (½ cup)	50	
Wheat Chex (¾ cup) + ½ cup skim milk + ½ banana	250	
Coffee	10	310 Cal
SNACK		
Fresh fruit in season (apple, plum, etc)	70	
Coffee or tea	10	80 Cal
LUNCH		
Soup (Appendix B - **page 118**)	90	
String cheese (1 piece, any brand)	80	
Whole-grain bread (1 slice)	70	
Coffee or tea	10	250 Cal
SNACK		
Handful unsalted mixed nuts	100	
Coffee or tea	10	110 Cal
DINNER		
Frozen Entrée (Appendix D - **page 122**)	320	
"Big-Bowl Salad"	150	
Whole-grain bread (1 slice)	70	
Fresh fruit in season (peach, pear, etc)	70	
Water with lemon wedge	15	625 Cal
SNACK		
Popcorn Mini Bag	110	
Coffee or tea	10	120 Cal
		1495 Cal

Day 39 1500 Calorie Meal Plan

BREAKFAST	Calories	Totals
Fresh or frozen strawberries (½ cup)	25	
Kashi Go Lean Waffles (2)	150	
Morningstar Breakfast Sausage Link	80	
Light Syrup (2 Tbsp)	50	
Coffee	10	315 Cal
SNACK		
Yogurt (4 oz, non-fat, any flavor)	60	
Coffee or tea	10	70 Cal
LUNCH		
Steak, Egg & Cheese*	280	
Fresh fruit in season (apple, plum, etc)	70	
Diet soda or water	0	350 Cal
* Hot Pockets (wrap)		
SNACK		
Handful unsalted mixed nuts	100	
Coffee or tea	10	110 Cal
DINNER		
Frozen Entrée (Appendix D - **page 122**)	260	
"Big-Bowl Salad"	150	
Whole-grain bread (1 slice)	70	
Hot or iced tea	10	490 Cal
SNACK		
Skinny Cow Ice Cream Sandwich	160	
Coffee or tea	10	170 Cal
		1505 Cal

Day 40 1500 Calorie Meal Plan

BREAKFAST	Calories	Totals
Grapefruit (½)	75	
Fried egg	80	
Whole-grain toast (1 slice)	70	
Coffee	10	235 Cal
SNACK		
Yogurt (4 oz, non-fat, any flavor)	60	
Coffee or tea	10	70 Cal
LUNCH		
Salad (3 oz canned tuna, 1 tsp Evoo, onions, celery)	175	
String cheese (1 piece, any brand - 80 Cal max)	80	
Rye bread (1 slice)	70	
Hot or iced tea	10	335 Cal
SNACK		
Handful unsalted mixed nuts	100	
Coffee or tea	10	110 Cal
DINNER		
Frozen Entrée (Appendix D - **page 122**)	330	
"Big-Bowl Salad"	150	
Whole-grain bread (1 slice)	70	
Fresh fruit in season (peach, plum, etc)	70	
Water	0	620 Cal
SNACK		
Popcorn Mini Bag	110	
Coffee or tea	10	120 Cal
		1490 Cal

Day 41 1500 Calorie Meal Plan

BREAKFAST	Calories	Totals
Fresh sliced orange	75	
Cheerios (1 cup) + ½ cup skim milk + about 15 raisins	190	
Whole-grain toast (1 slice)	70	
Coffee	10	345 Cal
SNACK		
Kashi TLC Chewy Granola Bar	140	
Coffee or tea	10	150 Cal
LUNCH		
Cottage cheese (1 cup low fat)	180	
Fresh fruit in season (apple, plum, etc)	70	
Small whole-grain roll	80	
Coffee or tea	10	340 Cal
SNACK		
Handful unsalted mixed nuts	100	
Coffee or tea	10	110 Cal
DINNER		
Frozen Entrée (Appendix D - **page 122**)	220	
"Big-Bowl Salad"	150	
Whole-grain bread (1 slice)	70	
Water	0	440 Cal
SNACK		
Popcorn Mini Bag	110	
Coffee or tea	10	120 Cal
		1505 Cal

Day 42 1500 Calorie Meal Plan

BREAKFAST	Calories	Totals
Grapefruit (½)	75	
Soft-boiled egg	80	
Turkey bacon (1 slice)	35	
Whole-grain toast (1 slice)	70	
Coffee	10	270 Cal
SNACK		
Fresh fruit in season (peach, plum, etc)	70	
Coffee or tea	10	80 Cal
LUNCH		
Soup (Appendix B - **page 118**)*	220	
Laughing Cow Light Cheese (1 wedge)	35	
Small whole-grain roll	80	
Coffee or tea	10	345 Cal
SNACK		
Yogurt (4 oz, non-fat, any flavor)	60	
Coffee or tea	10	70 Cal
DINNER		
Frozen Entrée (Appendix D - **page 122**)	340	
"Big-Bowl Salad"	150	
Fresh fruit in season (apple, plum, etc)	70	
Water with lemon wedge	15	575 Cal
SNACK		
Skinny Cow Ice Cream Sandwich	160	
Coffee or tea	10	170 Cal
		1510 Cal

Day 43 1500 Calorie Meal Plan		
BREAKFAST	Calories	Totals
Orange juice (½ cup)	50	
Shredded Wheat **(1 cup)** + **½ cup skim milk** + **½ banana**	260	
Coffee	10	320 Cal
SNACK		
Fresh fruit in season (peach, plum, etc)	70	
Coffee or tea	10	80 Cal
LUNCH		
Peanut butter (2 Tbsp) on 2 slices bread	340	
Skim milk (8 oz)	90	
Fresh fruit in season (apple, plum, etc)	70	
Water	0	500 Cal
SNACK		
Nature Valley Crunchy Granola bar	95	
Coffee or tea	10	105 Cal
DINNER		
Frozen Entrée (Appendix D **- page 122**)	180	
"Big-Bowl Salad"	150	
Whole-grain bread (1 slice)	70	
Diet soda or water	0	400 Cal
SNACK		
100-Calorie Pack Cookies	100	
Coffee or tea	10	110 Cal
		1515 Cal

Day 44 1500 Calorie Meal Plan		
BREAKFAST	Calories	Totals
Cantaloupe (½ medium)	50	
Oatmeal (**½ cup dry**) + ½ cup skim milk + **15 raisins**	220	
Coffee	10	280 Cal
SNACK		
Fresh fruit in season (apple, pear, etc)	70	
Coffee or tea	10	80 Cal
LUNCH		
Frozen Entrée (Appendix D **- page 122**)	350	
Diet soda or water	0	350 Cal
SNACK		
Yogurt (4 oz, non-fat, any flavor)	60	
Coffee or tea	10	70 Cal
DINNER		
Eat Out – Fish dinner		
– Maximum allowable calories	610	610 Cal
SNACK		
100-Calorie Pack Cookies	100	
Coffee or tea	10	110 Cal
		1500 Cal

Day 45 1200 Calorie Meal Plan

BREAKFAST	Calories	Totals
Fresh sliced orange	75	
Wheaties (¾ cup) + ½ cup skim milk + ½ banana	190	
Whole grain toast (1 slice)	70	
Coffee	10	345 Cal
SNACK		
Fresh fruit in season (apple, peach, etc)	70	
Coffee or tea	10	80 Cal
LUNCH		
Subway 6" (Ham, Cheese + veggies)*	260	
Water with lemon wedge	15	275 Cal
SNACK		
Handful unsalted mixed nuts	100	
Coffee or tea	10	110 Cal
DINNER		
Frozen Entrée (Appendix D - page 122)	340	
"Big-Bowl Salad"	150	
Fresh fruit in season (peach, plum, etc)	70	
Water with lemon wedge	15	575 Cal
SNACK		
Popcorn Mini Bag	110	
Coffee or tea	10	120 Cal
		1505 Cal

Day 46 1500 Calorie Meal Plan		
BREAKFAST	Calories	Totals
Orange juice (½ cup)	50	
Wheat Chex (¾ cup) + ½ cup skim milk + ½ banana	250	
Coffee	10	310 Cal
SNACK		
Yogurt (4 oz, non-fat, any flavor)	60	
Coffee or tea	10	70 Cal
LUNCH		
Steak, Egg & Cheese*	280	
Fresh fruit in season (peach, plum, etc)	70	
Diet soda or water	0	350 Cal
* Hot Pockets (wrap)		
SNACK		
Handful unsalted mixed nuts	100	
Coffee or tea	10	110 Cal
DINNER		
Frozen Entrée (Appendix D **- page 122**)	200	
"Big-Bowl Salad"	150	
Whole-grain bread (1 slice)	70	
Fresh fruit in season (pear, plum, etc)	70	
Water	0	490 Cal
SNACK		
Skinny Cow Ice Cream Sandwich	160	
Coffee or tea	10	170 Cal
		1500 Cal

Day 47 1500 Calorie Meal Plan

BREAKFAST	Calories	Totals
Cantaloupe (½ medium)	50	
Fried egg	80	
Turkey bacon (2 slices)	70	
Toasted raisin bread (1 slice)	75	
Coffee	10	285 Cal
SNACK		
Yogurt (4 oz, non-fat, any flavor)	60	
Coffee or tea	10	70 Cal
LUNCH		
Soup (Appendix B **- page 118**)	160	
String cheese (1 piece, any brand)	80	
Nature Valley Crunchy Granola bar	95	
Coffee or tea	10	345 Cal
SNACK		
Handful unsalted mixed nuts	100	
Coffee or tea	10	110 Cal
DINNER		
Frozen Entrée (Appendix D **- page 122**)	260	
"Big-Bowl Salad"	150	
Whole-grain bread (1 slice)	70	
Fresh fruit in season (apple, peach, etc)	70	
Water with lemon wedge	15	565 Cal
SNACK		
Popcorn Mini Bag	110	
Coffee or tea	10	120 Cal
		1495 Cal

Day 48 1500 Calorie Meal Plan		
BREAKFAST	Calories	Totals
Grapefruit (½)	75	
Cheerios (1 cup) + ½ cup skim milk + about 15 raisins	190	
Coffee	10	275 Cal
SNACK		
Kashi TLC Chewy Granola Bar	140	
Coffee or tea	10	150 Cal
LUNCH		
Cottage cheese (1 cup low fat)	180	
Fresh fruit in season (apple, plum, etc)	70	
Small whole-grain roll	80	
Coffee or tea	10	340 Cal
SNACK		
Handful unsalted mixed nuts	100	
Coffee or tea	10	110 Cal
DINNER		
Frozen Entrée (Appendix D **- page 122**)	220	
"Big-Bowl Salad"	150	
Whole-grain bread (1 slice)	70	
Fresh fruit in season (peach, plum, etc)	70	
Water	0	510 Cal
SNACK		
Popcorn Mini Bag	110	
Coffee or tea	10	120 Cal
		1505 Cal

Day 49 1500 Calorie Meal Plan

BREAKFAST	Calories	Totals
Grapefruit (½)	75	
Scrambled egg	80	
Whole-grain toast (1 slice)	70	
Coffee	10	235 Cal
SNACK		
Yogurt (4 oz, non-fat, any flavor)	60	
Coffee or tea	10	70 Cal
LUNCH		
Salad (3 oz canned tuna, 1 tsp Evoo, onions, celery)	175	
String cheese (1 piece, any brand - 80 Cal max)	80	
Rye bread (1 slice)	70	
Hot or iced tea	10	335 Cal
SNACK		
Handful unsalted mixed nuts	100	
Coffee or tea	10	110 Cal
DINNER		
Frozen Entrée (Appendix D **- page 122**)	350	
"Big-Bowl Salad"	150	
Fresh fruit in season (apple, pear, etc)	70	
Diet soda or water	0	570 Cal
SNACK		
Skinny Cow Ice Cream Sandwich	160	
Coffee or tea	10	170 Cal
		1490 Cal

Day 50 1500 Calorie Meal Plan		
BREAKFAST	Calories	Totals
Tomato juice (½ cup)	20	
Shredded Wheat **(1 cup)** + ½ **cup skim milk** + ½ **banana**	260	
Coffee	10	290 Cal
SNACK		
Yogurt (4 oz, non-fat, any flavor)	60	
Coffee or tea	10	70 Cal
LUNCH		
Subway 6" (Roast beef, Cheese + veggies)*	245	
Fresh fruit in season (apple, peach, etc)	70	
Water with lemon wedge	15	330 Cal
* **Half 9-grain roll.**		
SNACK		
Handful unsalted mixed nuts	100	
Coffee or tea	10	110 Cal
DINNER		
Frozen Entrée (Appendix D **- page 122**)	270	
"Big-Bowl Salad"	150	
Whole-grain bread (1 slice)	70	
Fresh fruit in season (peach, plum, etc)	70	
Water	0	560 Cal
SNACK		
Kashi TLC Chewy Granola Bar	140	140 Cal
		1500 Cal

Day 51 1500 Calorie Meal Plan

BREAKFAST	Calories	Totals
Cantaloupe (½ medium)	50	
Oatmeal (**½ cup dry**) + **½ cup skim milk** + **15 raisins**	220	
Coffee	10	280 Cal
SNACK		
Fresh fruit in season (apple, plum, etc)	70	
Coffee or tea	10	80 Cal
LUNCH		
Frozen Entrée (Appendix D **- page 122**)	290	
Diet soda or water	0	290 Cal
SNACK		
Yogurt (4 oz, non-fat, any flavor)	60	
Coffee or tea	10	70 Cal
DINNER		
Eat Out – Fish dinner		
– Maximum allowable calories	670	670 Cal
SNACK		
100-Calorie Pack Cookies	100	
Coffee or tea	10	110 Cal
		1500 Cal

Day 52 1500 Calorie Meal Plan		
BREAKFAST	Calories	Totals
Cantaloupe (½ medium)	50	
Wheat Chex (¾ cup) + ½ cup skim milk + ½ banana	250	
Coffee	10	310 Cal
SNACK		
Fresh fruit in season (peach, plum, etc)	70	
Coffee or tea	10	80 Cal
LUNCH		
Soup (Appendix B **- page 118**)	140	
String cheese (1 piece, any brand)	80	
Small whole-grain roll	80	
Coffee or tea	10	310 Cal
SNACK		
Handful unsalted mixed nuts	100	
Coffee or tea	10	110 Cal
DINNER		
Frozen Entrée (Appendix D **- page 122**)	270	
"Big-Bowl Salad"	150	
Whole-grain bread (1 slice)	70	
Fresh fruit in season (apple, plum, etc)	70	
Water with lemon wedge	15	575 Cal
SNACK		
Popcorn Mini Bag	110	
Coffee or tea	10	120 Cal
		1505 Cal

Day 53 1500 Calorie Meal Plan

BREAKFAST	Calories	Totals
Fresh or frozen strawberries (½ cup)	25	
Kashi Go Lean Waffles (2)	150	
Morningstar Breakfast Sausage Link	80	
Light Syrup (2 Tbsp)	50	
Coffee	10	315 Cal
SNACK		
Yogurt (4 oz, non-fat, any flavor)	60	
Coffee or tea	10	70 Cal
LUNCH		
Ham (2 oz) with mustard on 2 slices rye bread	300	
Pickle spear	0	
Fresh fruit in season (apple, peach, etc)	70	
Hot or iced tea	10	380 Cal
SNACK		
Handful unsalted mixed nuts	100	
Coffee or tea	10	110 Cal
DINNER		
Frozen Entrée (Appendix D - **page 122**)	230	
"Big-Bowl Salad"	150	
Fresh fruit in season (pear, plum, etc)	70	
Hot or iced tea	10	460 Cal
SNACK		
Skinny Cow Ice Cream Sandwich	160	
Coffee or tea	10	170 Cal
		1505 Cal

Day 54 1500 Calorie Meal Plan

BREAKFAST	Calories	Totals
Orange juice (½ cup)	50	
Fried egg	80	
Whole-grain toast (1 slice)	70	
Coffee	10	210 Cal
SNACK		
Fresh fruit in season (apple, pear, etc)	70	
Coffee or tea	10	80 Cal
LUNCH		
Soup (Appendix B - **page 118**)*	260	
String cheese (1 piece, any brand)	80	
Small whole-grain roll	80	
Coffee or tea	10	430 Cal
* **Enjoy 2 servings of 130 Cal soup.**		
SNACK		
Yogurt (4 oz, non-fat, any flavor)	60	
Coffee or tea	10	70 Cal
DINNER		
Frozen Entrée (Appendix D - **page 122**)	250	
"Big-Bowl Salad"	150	
Whole-grain bread (1 slice)	70	
Fresh fruit in season (peach, plum, etc)	70	
Water	0	540 Cal
SNACK		
Skinny Cow Ice Cream Sandwich	160	
Coffee or tea	10	170 Cal
		1500 Cal

Day 55 1500 Calorie Meal Plan		
BREAKFAST	Calories	Totals
Grapefruit (½)	75	
Cheerios (1 cup) + ½ cup skim milk + about 15 raisins	190	
Coffee	10	275 Cal
SNACK		
Handful unsalted mixed nuts	100	
Coffee or tea	10	110 Cal
LUNCH		
Cottage cheese (1 cup low fat)	180	
Fresh fruit in season (apple, pear, etc)	70	
Whole-grain bread (1 slice)	70	
Coffee or tea	10	330 Cal
SNACK		
Kashi TLC Chewy Granola Bar	140	
Coffee or tea	10	150 Cal
DINNER		
Frozen Entrée (Appendix D **- page 122**)	280	
"Big-Bowl Salad"	150	
Small whole-grain roll	80	
Water	0	510 Cal
SNACK		
Popcorn Mini Bag	110	
Coffee or tea	10	120 Cal
		1495 Cal

Day 56 1500 Calorie Meal Plan		
BREAKFAST	Calories	Totals
Cantaloupe (½ medium)	50	
Soft-boiled egg	80	
Toasted whole-grain bread (1 slice)	70	
Coffee	10	210 Cal
SNACK		
Yogurt (4 oz, non-fat, any flavor)	60	
Coffee or tea	10	70 Cal
LUNCH		
Subway 6" (Turkey, Cheese + veggies)*	230	
Fresh fruit in season (peach, plum, etc)	70	
Water with lemon wedge	15	315 Cal
* Half 9-grain roll.		
SNACK		
Handful unsalted mixed nuts	100	
Coffee or tea	10	110 Cal
DINNER		
Frozen Entrée (Appendix D **- page 122**)	310	
"Big-Bowl Salad"	150	
Whole-grain bread (1 slice)	70	
Fresh fruit in season (apple, pear, etc)	70	
Water with lemon wedge	15	615 Cal
SNACK		
Skinny Cow Ice Cream Sandwich	160	
Coffee or tea	10	170 Cal
		1490 Cal

Day 57 1500 Calorie Meal Plan

BREAKFAST	Calories	Totals
Cantaloupe (½ medium)	50	
Oatmeal (**½ cup dry**) + **½ cup skim milk** + **15 raisins**	220	
Coffee	10	280 Cal
SNACK		
Yogurt (4 oz, non-fat, any flavor)	60	
Coffee or tea	10	70 Cal
LUNCH		
Chicken Pot Pie*	230	
Fresh fruit in season (apple, plum, etc)	70	
Hot or iced tea	10	310 Cal
* Hot Pockets (wrap)		
SNACK		
Handful unsalted mixed nuts	100	
Coffee or tea	10	110 Cal
DINNER		
Frozen Entrée (Appendix D **- page 122**)	290	
"Big-Bowl Salad"	150	
Whole-grain bread (1 slice)	70	
Fresh fruit in season (pear, plum, etc)	70	
Water	0	580 Cal
SNACK		
Kashi TLC Chewy Granola Bar	140	
Coffee or tea	10	150 Cal
		1500 Cal

Day 58 1500 Calorie Meal Plan

BREAKFAST	Calories	Totals
Tomato juice (½ cup)	20	
Shredded Wheat **(1 cup) + ½ cup skim milk + ½ banana**	260	
Coffee	10	290 Cal
SNACK		
Fresh fruit in season (apple, plum, etc)	70	
Coffee or tea	10	80 Cal
LUNCH		
Subway 6" (Roast Beef, Cheese + veggies)	245	
Diet soda (or water)	0	245 Cal
SNACK		
Yogurt (4 oz, non-fat, any flavor)	60	
Coffee or tea	10	70 Cal
DINNER		
Eat Out – Fish dinner		
– Maximum allowable calories	670	670 Cal
SNACK		
Kashi TLC Chewy Granola Bar	140	
Coffee or tea	10	150 Cal
		1505 Cal

Day 59 1500 Calorie Meal Plan

BREAKFAST	Calories	Totals
Orange juice (½ cup)	50	
Wheaties (¾ cup) + ½ cup skim milk + ½ banana	190	
Whole-grain toast (1 slice)	70	
Coffee	10	320 Cal
SNACK		
Fresh fruit in season (apple, plum, etc)	70	
Coffee or tea	10	80 Cal
LUNCH		
Salad (3 oz canned tuna, 1 tsp Evoo, onions, celery)	175	
String cheese (1 piece, any brand - 80 Cal max)	80	
Rye bread (1 slice)	70	
Diet soda or water	0	325 Cal
SNACK		
Handful unsalted mixed nuts	100	
Coffee or tea	10	110 Cal
DINNER		
Frozen Entrée (Appendix D - **page 122**)	250	
"Big-Bowl Salad"	150	
Whole-grain bread (1 slice)	70	
Fresh fruit in season (peach, plum, etc)	70	
Water	15	520 Cal
SNACK		
Popcorn Mini Bag	110	
Coffee or tea	10	120 Cal
		1495 Cal

Day 60 1500 Calorie Meal Plan		
BREAKFAST	Calories	Totals
Orange juice (½ cup)	50	
Kashi Go Lean Waffles (2)	150	
Morningstar Breakfast Sausage Link	80	
Light Syrup (2 Tbsp)	50	
Coffee	10	340 Cal
SNACK		
Yogurt (4 oz, non-fat, any flavor)	60	
Coffee or tea	10	70 Cal
LUNCH		
Chicken, Broccoli & Cheese*	260	
Fresh fruit in season (peach, plum, etc)	70	
Diet soda or water	10	340 Cal
* Hot Pockets (wrap)		
SNACK		
Handful unsalted mixed nuts	100	
Coffee or tea	10	110 Cal
DINNER		
Frozen Entrée (Appendix D - **page 122**)	180	
"Big-Bowl Salad"	150	
Whole-grain bread (1 slice)	70	
Fresh fruit in season (apple, plum, etc)	70	
Water	0	470 Cal
SNACK		
Skinny Cow Ice Cream Sandwich	160	
Coffee or tea	10	170 Cal
		1500 Cal

Day 61 1500 Calorie Meal Plan

BREAKFAST	Calories	Totals
Orange juice (½ cup)	50	
Wheaties (¾ cup) + ½ cup skim milk + ½ banana	190	
Whole-grain toast (1 slice)	70	
Coffee	10	320 Cal
SNACK		
Handful unsalted mixed nuts	100	
Coffee or tea	10	110 Cal
LUNCH		
Soup (Appendix B - page 118)	110	
Whole-grain bread (1 slice)	70	
Coffee or tea	10	190 Cal
SNACK		
100-Calorie Pack Cookies	100	
Coffee or tea	10	110 Cal
DINNER		
Frozen Entrée (Appendix D - page 122)	310	
"Big-Bowl Salad"	150	
Whole grain bread (1 slice)	70	
Fresh fruit in season (apple, pear, etc)	70	
Water with lemon wedge	15	615 Cal
SNACK		
Kashi TLC Chewy Granola Bar	140	
Coffee or tea	10	150 Cal
		1495 Cal

Day 62 1500 Calorie Meal Plan

BREAKFAST	Calories	Totals
Fresh or frozen strawberries (½ cup)	25	
Kashi Go Lean Waffles (2)	150	
Morningstar Breakfast Sausage Link	80	
Light Syrup (2 Tbsp)	50	
Coffee	10	315 Cal
SNACK		
Handful unsalted mixed nuts	100	
Coffee or tea	10	110 Cal
LUNCH		
Ham (2 oz) with mustard on 2 slices rye bread	300	
Laughing Cow Light Cheese (1 wedge)	35	
Fresh fruit in season (apple, peach, etc)	70	
Coffee or tea	10	415 Cal
SNACK		
Kashi TLC Chewy Granola Bar	140	
Coffee or tea	10	150 Cal
DINNER		
Frozen Entrée (Appendix D - **page 122**)	180	
"Big-Bowl Salad"	150	
Water with lemon wedge	15	345 Cal
SNACK		
Skinny Cow Ice Cream Sandwich	160	
Coffee or tea	10	170 Cal
		1505 Cal

Day 63 1500 Calorie Meal Plan

BREAKFAST	Calories	Totals
Grapefruit (½)	75	
Fried egg	80	
Whole-grain toast (2 slices)	140	
Coffee	10	305 Cal
SNACK		
Handful unsalted mixed nuts	100	
Coffee or tea	10	110 Cal
LUNCH		
Soup (Appendix B - **page 118**)	140	
String cheese (1 piece, any brand)	80	
Fresh fruit in season (pear, peach, etc)	70	
Water	0	290 Cal
SNACK		
Kashi TLC Chewy Granola Bar	140	
Coffee or tea	10	150 Cal
DINNER		
Frozen Entrée (Appendix D - **page 122**)	240	
"Big-Bowl Salad"	150	
Whole-grain bread (1 slice)	70	
Water with lemon wedge	15	475 Cal
SNACK		
Skinny Cow Ice Cream Sandwich	160	
Coffee or tea	10	170 Cal
		1500 Cal

Day 64 1500 Calorie Meal Plan

BREAKFAST	Calories	Totals
Grapefruit (½)	75	
Scrambled egg (1)	80	
Turkey bacon (1 slice)	35	
Whole grain toast (1 slice)	70	
Coffee	10	270 Cal
SNACK		
Yogurt (4 oz, non-fat, any flavor)	60	
Coffee or tea	10	70 Cal
LUNCH		
Subway 6" (**Turkey breast, Cheese + veggies**)	230	
Fresh fruit in season (apple, plum, etc)	70	
Diet soda or water	0	300 Cal
SNACK		
Handful unsalted mixed nuts	100	
Coffee or tea	10	110 Cal
DINNER		
Frozen Entrée (Appendix D)	270	
"Big-Bowl Salad"	150	
Whole-grain bread (1 slice)	70	
Fresh fruit in season (apple, peach, etc)	70	
Water	0	560 Cal
SNACK		
Kashi TLC Crunchy Granola Bar	180	
Coffee or tea	10	190 Cal
		1500 Cal

Day 65 1500 Calorie Meal Plan		
BREAKFAST	Calories	Totals
Cantaloupe (½ medium)	50	
Fried egg	80	
Toasted whole-grain bread (1 slice)	70	
Coffee	10	210 Cal
SNACK		
Yogurt (4 oz, non-fat, any flavor)	60	
Coffee or tea	10	70 Cal
LUNCH		
Soup (Appendix B - **page 118**)*	260	
String cheese (1 piece, any brand)	80	
Fresh fruit in season (apple, peach, etc)	80	
Coffee or tea	10	430 Cal
* Enjoy 2 servings of 130 Cal soup.		
SNACK		
Handful unsalted mixed nuts	100	
Coffee or tea	10	110 Cal
DINNER		
Frozen Entrée (Appendix D - **page 122**)	240	
"Big-Bowl Salad"	150	
Whole-grain bread (1 slice)	70	
Fresh fruit in season (peach, plum, etc)	70	
Water	0	530 Cal
SNACK		
Skinny Cow Ice Cream Sandwich	160	
Coffee or tea	10	170 Cal
		1510 Cal

Day 66 1500 Calorie Meal Plan		
BREAKFAST	Calories	Totals
Tomato juice (½ cup)	20	
Shredded Wheat **(1 cup)** + **½ cup skim milk** + **½ banana**	265	
Coffee	10	295 Cal
SNACK		
Yogurt (4 oz, non-fat, any flavor)	60	
Coffee or tea	10	70 Cal
LUNCH		
Chicken, Bacon Ranch*	270	
Fresh fruit in season (apple, plum, etc)	70	
Hot or iced tea	10	350 Cal
* Hot Pockets (wrap)		
SNACK		
Handful unsalted mixed nuts	100	
Coffee or tea	10	110 Cal
DINNER		
Frozen Entrée (Appendix D - **page 122**)	340	
"Big-Bowl Salad"	150	
Whole-grain bread (1 slice)	70	
Water with lemon wedge	15	575 Cal
SNACK		
Nature Valley Crunchy Granola bar	95	
Coffee or tea	10	105 Cal
		1505 Cal

Day 67 1500 Calorie Meal Plan		
BREAKFAST	Calories	Totals
Cantaloupe (½ medium)	50	
Oatmeal (½ cup dry) + ½ cup skim milk + 15 raisins	220	
Coffee	10	280 Cal
SNACK		
Fresh fruit in season (apple, plum, etc)	70	
Coffee or tea	10	80 Cal
LUNCH		
Frozen Entrée (Appendix D - page 122)	290	
Diet soda or water	0	290 Cal
SNACK		
Yogurt (4 oz, non-fat, any flavor)	60	
Coffee or tea	10	70 Cal
DINNER		
Eat Out – Fish dinner		
– Maximum allowable calories	670	670 Cal
SNACK		
100-Calorie Pack Cookies	100	
Coffee or tea	10	110 Cal
		1500 Cal

Day 68 1500 Calorie Meal Plan		
BREAKFAST	Calories	Totals
Orange juice (½ cup)	50	
Wheat Chex (¾ cup) + ½ cup skim milk + ½ banana	250	
Coffee	10	310 Cal
SNACK		
Fresh fruit in season (peach, plum, etc)	70	
Coffee or tea	10	80 Cal
LUNCH		
Soup (Appendix B **- page 118**)	100	
String cheese (1 piece, any brand)	80	
Whole-grain bread (1 slice)	70	
Coffee or tea	10	260 Cal
SNACK		
Handful unsalted mixed nuts	100	
Coffee or tea	10	110 Cal
DINNER		
Frozen Entrée (Appendix D **- page 122**)	320	
"Big-Bowl Salad"	150	
Whole-grain bread (1 slice)	70	
Fresh fruit in season (pear, plum, etc)	70	
Hot or iced tea	10	620 Cal
SNACK		
Popcorn Mini Bag	110	
Coffee or tea	10	120 Cal
		1500 Cal

Day 69 1500 Calorie Meal Plan

BREAKFAST	Calories	Totals
Fresh or frozen strawberries (½ cup)	25	
Kashi Go Lean Waffles (2)	150	
Morningstar Breakfast Sausage Link	80	
Light Syrup (2 Tbsp)	50	
Coffee	10	315 Cal
SNACK		
Yogurt (4 oz, non-fat, any flavor)	60	
Coffee or tea	10	70 Cal
LUNCH		
Chorizo, Egg & Cheese*	260	
Fresh fruit in season (apple, plum, etc)	70	
Hot or iced tea	10	340 Cal
* Hot Pockets (wrap)		
SNACK		
Handful unsalted mixed nuts	100	
Coffee or tea	10	110 Cal
DINNER		
Frozen Entrée (Appendix D **- page 122**)	270	
"Big-Bowl Salad"	150	
Whole-grain bread (1 slice)	70	
Water with lemon wedge	15	505 Cal
SNACK		
Skinny Cow Ice Cream Sandwich	160	
Coffee or tea	10	170 Cal
		1510 Cal

Day 70 1500 Calorie Meal Plan

BREAKFAST	Calories	Totals
Grapefruit (½)	75	
Soft-boiled egg	80	
Whole-grain toast (1 slice)	70	
Coffee	10	235 Cal
SNACK		
Yogurt (4 oz, non-fat, any flavor)	60	
Coffee or tea	10	70 Cal
LUNCH		
Salad (3 oz canned tuna, 1 tsp Evoo, onions, celery)	175	
Rye bread (1 slice)	70	
Laughing Cow Light Cheese (1 wedge)	35	
Small bunch of grapes	65	
Coffee or tea	10	355 Cal
SNACK		
Handful unsalted mixed nuts	100	
Coffee or tea	10	110 Cal
DINNER		
Frozen Entrée (Appendix D - **page 122**)	300	
"Big-Bowl Salad"	150	
Whole-grain bread (1 slice)	70	
Fresh fruit in season (pear, plum, etc)	70	
Water with lemon wedge	15	605 Cal
SNACK		
Popcorn Mini Bag	110	
Coffee or tea	10	120 Cal
		1495 Cal

Day 71 1500 Calorie Meal Plan

BREAKFAST	Calories	Totals
Fresh sliced orange	75	
Cheerios (1 cup) + ½ cup skim milk + about 15 raisins	190	
Whole-grain toast (1 slice)	70	
Coffee	10	345 Cal
SNACK		
Kashi TLC Chewy Granola Bar	140	140 Cal
LUNCH		
Subway 6" (Roast beef, Cheese + veggies)*	245	
Fresh fruit in season (apple, plum, etc)	70	
Hot or iced tea	10	325 Cal
SNACK		
Handful unsalted mixed nuts	100	
Coffee or tea	10	110 Cal
DINNER		
Frozen Entrée (Appendix D - **page 122**)	250	
"Big-Bowl Salad"	150	
Whole-grain bread (1 slice)	70	
Water	0	470 Cal
SNACK		
100-Calorie Pack Cookies	100	
Coffee or tea	10	110 Cal
		1500 Cal

Day 72 1500 Calorie Meal Plan

BREAKFAST	Calories	Totals
Grapefruit (½)	75	
Scrambled egg	80	
Turkey bacon (1 slice)	35	
Whole-grain toast (1 slice)	70	
Coffee	10	270 Cal
SNACK		
Fresh fruit in season (peach, plum, etc)	70	
Coffee or tea	10	80 Cal
LUNCH		
Soup (Appendix B - **page 118**)*	260	
Laughing Cow Light Cheese (1 wedge)	35	
Small whole-grain roll	80	
Coffee or tea	10	385 Cal
* Enjoy 2 servings of 130 Cal soup.		
SNACK		
Yogurt (4 oz, non-fat, any flavor)	60	
Coffee or tea	10	70 Cal
DINNER		
Frozen Entrée (Appendix D - **page 122**)	300	
"Big-Bowl Salad"	150	
Fresh fruit in season (apple, peach, etc)	70	
Water	0	520 Cal
SNACK		
Skinny Cow Ice Cream Sandwich	160	
Coffee or tea	10	170 Cal
		1495 Cal

Day 73 1500 Calorie Meal Plan		
BREAKFAST	Calories	Totals
Tomato juice (½ cup)	20	
Shredded Wheat **(1 cup)** + **½ cup skim milk** + **½ banana**	265	
Whole-grain toast (1 slice)	70	
Coffee	10	365 Cal
SNACK		
Yogurt (4 oz, non-fat, any flavor)	60	
Coffee or tea	10	70 Cal
LUNCH		
Chicken Pot Pie*	230	
Fresh fruit in season (apple, plum, etc)	70	
Hot or iced tea	10	310 Cal
* Hot Pockets (wrap)		
SNACK		
Handful unsalted mixed nuts	100	
Coffee or tea	10	110 Cal
DINNER		
Frozen Entrée (Appendix D **- page 122**)	180	
"Big-Bowl Salad"	150	
Whole-grain bread (1 slice)	70	
Fresh blueberries, cherries or grapes (1 cup)	100	
Water	0	500 Cal
SNACK		
Kashi TLC Chewy Granola Bar	140	
Coffee or tea	10	150 Cal
		1505 Cal

Day 74 1500 Calorie Meal Plan

BREAKFAST	Calories	Totals
Cantaloupe (½ medium)	50	
Oatmeal (**½ cup dry**) + **½ cup skim milk** + **15 raisins**	220	
Coffee	10	280 Cal
SNACK		
Fresh fruit in season (apple, peach, etc)	70	
Coffee or tea	10	80 Cal
LUNCH		
Frozen Entrée (Appendix D **- page 122**)	290	
Diet soda or water	0	290 Cal
SNACK		
Yogurt (4 oz, non-fat, any flavor)	60	
Coffee or tea	10	70 Cal
DINNER		
Eat Out – Fish dinner		
– Maximum allowable calories	670	670 Cal
SNACK		
100-Calorie Pack Cookies	100	
Coffee or tea	10	110 Cal
		1500 Cal

Day 75 1500 Calorie Meal Plan

BREAKFAST	Calories	Totals
Fresh sliced orange	75	
Wheaties (¾ cup) + ½ cup skim milk + ½ banana	190	
Toasted raisin bread (1 slice)	75	
Coffee	10	350 Cal
SNACK		
Fresh fruit in season (apple, peach, etc)	70	
Coffee or tea	10	80 Cal
LUNCH		
Soup (Appendix B - **page 118**)	100	
String cheese (1 piece, any brand)	80	
Small whole-grain roll	80	
Coffee or tea	10	270 Cal
SNACK		
Handful unsalted mixed nuts	100	
Coffee or tea	10	110 Cal
DINNER		
Frozen Entrée (Appendix D - **page 122**)	330	
"Big-Bowl Salad"	150	
Fresh fruit in season (apple, plum, etc)	70	
Hot or iced tea	10	550 Cal
SNACK		
Popcorn Mini Bag	110	
Coffee or tea	10	120 Cal
		1500 Cal

Day 76 1500 Calorie Meal Plan		
BREAKFAST	Calories	Totals
Orange juice (½ cup)	50	
Wheat Chex (¾ cup) + ½ cup skim milk + ½ banana	250	
Coffee	10	310 Cal
SNACK		
Yogurt (4 oz, non-fat, any flavor)	60	
Coffee or tea	10	70 Cal
LUNCH		
Ham & Cheddar*	270	
Fresh fruit in season (peach, plum, etc)	70	
Diet soda or water	0	340 Cal
* Hot Pockets (wrap)		
SNACK		
Handful unsalted mixed nuts	100	
Coffee or tea	10	110 Cal
DINNER		
Frozen Entrée (Appendix D **- page 122**)	200	
"Big-Bowl Salad"	150	
Whole-grain bread (1 slice)	70	
Fresh fruit in season (pear, plum, etc)	70	
Water	0	500 Cal
SNACK		
Skinny Cow Ice Cream Sandwich	160	
Coffee or tea	10	170 Cal
		1500 Cal

Day 77 1500 Calorie Meal Plan		
BREAKFAST	Calories	Totals
Cantaloupe (½ medium)	50	
Scrambled egg	80	
Toasted raisin bread (1 slice)	75	
Coffee	10	215 Cal
SNACK		
Yogurt (4 oz, non-fat, any flavor)	60	
Coffee or tea	10	70 Cal
LUNCH		
Soup (Appendix B - **page 118**)	160	
Whole-grain bread (1 slice)	70	
Banana (1 medium)	100	
Hot or iced tea	10	340 Cal
SNACK		
Fresh fruit in season (apple, plum, etc)	70	
Coffee or tea	10	80 Cal
DINNER		
Frozen Entrée (Appendix D - **page 122**)	290	
"Big-Bowl Salad"	150	
Small whole-grain roll	80	
Glass of wine (4 oz)	100	
Water with lemon wedge	15	635 Cal
SNACK		
Skinny Cow Ice Cream Sandwich	160	
Coffee or tea	10	170 Cal
		1510 Cal

Day 78 1500 Calorie Meal Plan

BREAKFAST	Calories	Totals
Grapefruit (½)	75	
Cheerios (1 cup) + ½ cup skim milk + about 15 raisins	190	
Coffee	10	275 Cal
SNACK		
Kashi TLC Chewy Granola Bar	140	
Coffee or tea	10	150 Cal
LUNCH		
Cottage cheese (1 cup low fat)	180	
Fresh fruit in season (pear, plum, etc)	70	
Small whole-grain roll	80	
Coffee or tea	10	340 Cal
SNACK		
Handful unsalted mixed nuts	100	
Coffee or tea	10	110 Cal
DINNER		
Frozen Entrée (Appendix D **- page 122**)	220	
"Big-Bowl Salad"	150	
Whole-grain bread (1 slice)	70	
Fresh fruit in season (apple, plum, etc)	70	
Water	0	510 Cal
SNACK		
Popcorn Mini Bag	110	
Coffee or tea	10	120 Cal
		1505 Cal

Day 79 1500 Calorie Meal Plan

BREAKFAST	Calories	Totals
Grapefruit (½)	75	
Fried egg	80	
Turkey bacon (1 slice)	35	
Whole-grain toast (1 slice)	70	
Coffee	10	270 Cal
SNACK		
Yogurt (4 oz, non-fat, any flavor)	60	
Coffee or tea	10	70 Cal
LUNCH		
Subway 6" (Ham, Cheese + veggies)	260	
Fresh fruit in season (apple, peach, etc)	70	
Diet soda or water	0	330 Cal
SNACK		
Handful unsalted mixed nuts	100	
Coffee or tea	10	110 Cal
DINNER		
Frozen Entrée (Appendix D - **page 122**)	340	
"Big-Bowl Salad"	150	
Fresh fruit in season (pear, peach, etc)	70	
Hot or iced tea	10	570 Cal
SNACK		
Kashi TLC Chewy Granola Bar	140	
Coffee or tea	10	150 Cal
		1500 Cal

Day 80 1500 Calorie Meal Plan

BREAKFAST	Calories	Totals
Tomato juice (½ cup)	20	
Shredded Wheat **(1 cup) + ½ cup skim milk + ½ banana**	265	
Coffee	10	295 Cal
SNACK		
Handful unsalted mixed nuts	100	
Coffee or tea	10	110 Cal
LUNCH		
Chorizo, Egg & Cheese*	260	
Fresh fruit in season (apple, plum, etc)	70	
Diet soda or water	0	330 Cal
* Hot Pockets (wrap)		
SNACK		
Yogurt (4 oz, non-fat, any flavor)	60	
Coffee or tea	10	70 Cal
DINNER		
Frozen Entrée (Appendix D **- page 122**)	230	
"Big-Bowl Salad"	150	
Whole-grain bread (1 slice)	70	
Fresh blueberries, cherries or grapes (1 cup)	100	
Water	0	550 Cal
SNACK		
Kashi TLC Chewy Granola Bar	140	
Coffee or tea	10	150 Cal
		1505 Cal

Day 81 1500 Calorie Meal Plan

BREAKFAST	Calories	Totals
Cantaloupe (½ medium)	50	
Oatmeal (½ **cup dry**) + ½ **cup skim milk** + **15 raisins**	220	
Coffee	10	280 Cal
SNACK		
Fresh fruit in season (pear, plum, etc)	70	
Coffee or tea	10	80 Cal
LUNCH		
Frozen Entrée (Appendix D **- page 122**)	290	
Diet soda or water	0	290 Cal
SNACK		
Yogurt (4 oz, non-fat, any flavor)	60	
Coffee or tea	10	70 Cal
DINNER		
Eat Out – Fish dinner		
– Maximum allowable calories	670	670 Cal
SNACK		
Popcorn Mini Bag	110	
Coffee or tea	10	120 Cal
		1510 Cal

Day 82 1500 Calorie Meal Plan		
BREAKFAST	Calories	Totals
Orange juice (½ cup)	50	
Wheat Chex (¾ cup) + ½ cup skim milk + ½ banana	250	
Coffee	10	310 Cal
SNACK		
Fresh fruit in season (peach, plum, etc)	70	
Coffee or tea	10	80 Cal
LUNCH		
Soup (Appendix B - **page 118**)	140	
String cheese (1 piece, any brand)	80	
Whole-grain bread (1 slice)	70	
Coffee or tea	10	300 Cal
SNACK		
Handful unsalted mixed nuts	100	
Coffee or tea	10	110 Cal
DINNER		
Frozen Entrée (Appendix D - **page 122**)	250	
"Big-Bowl Salad"	150	
Whole-grain bread (1 slice)	70	
Fresh fruit in season (apple, peach, etc)	70	
Water with lemon wedge	15	555 Cal
SNACK		
Kashi TLC Chewy Granola Bar	140	140 Cal
		1495 Cal

Day 83 1500 Calorie Meal Plan

BREAKFAST	Calories	Totals
Orange juice (½ cup)	50	
Kashi Go Lean Waffles (2)	150	
Morningstar Breakfast Sausage Link	80	
Light Syrup (2 Tbsp)	50	
Coffee	10	340 Cal
SNACK		
Yogurt (4 oz, non-fat, any flavor)	60	
Coffee or tea	10	70 Cal
LUNCH		
Southwest-Style Taco*	270	
Fresh fruit in season (apple, plum, etc)	70	
Diet soda or water	0	340 Cal
* Hot Pockets (wrap)		
SNACK		
Popcorn Mini Bag	110	
Coffee or tea	10	120 Cal
DINNER		
Frozen Entrée (Appendix D - **page 122**)	240	
"Big-Bowl Salad"	150	
Whole-grain bread (1 slice)	70	
Water	0	460 Cal
SNACK		
Skinny Cow Ice Cream Sandwich	160	
Coffee or tea	10	170 Cal
		1500 Cal

Day 84 1500 Calorie Meal Plan		
BREAKFAST	Calories	Totals
Orange juice (½ cup)	50	
Soft-boiled egg	80	
Whole-grain toast (1 slice)	70	
Coffee	10	210 Cal
SNACK		
Fresh fruit in season (apple, plum, etc)	70	
Coffee or tea	10	80 Cal
LUNCH		
Soup (Appendix B - **page 118**)*	260	
Small whole-grain roll	80	
Nature Valley Crunchy Granola bar	95	
Coffee or tea	10	445 Cal
* Enjoy 2 servings of 130 Cal soup.		
SNACK		
Yogurt (4 oz, non-fat, any flavor)	60	
Coffee or tea	10	70 Cal
DINNER		
Frozen Entrée (Appendix D - **page 122**)	250	
"Big-Bowl Salad"	150	
Whole-grain bread (1 slice)	70	
Fresh fruit in season (apple, peach, plum, etc)	70	
Water	0	540 Cal
SNACK		
Skinny Cow Ice Cream Sandwich	160	
Coffee or tea	10	170 Cal
		1515 Cal

Day 85 1500 Calorie Meal Plan

BREAKFAST	Calories	Totals
Grapefruit (½)	75	
Cheerios (1 cup) + ½ cup skim milk + about 15 raisins	190	
Coffee	10	275 Cal
SNACK		
Handful unsalted mixed nuts	100	
Coffee or tea	10	110 Cal
LUNCH		
Subway 6" (**Roast Beef, Cheese + veggies**)	245	
Fresh fruit in season (apple, plum, etc)	70	
Diet soda or water	0	315 Cal
SNACK		
Kashi TLC Chewy Granola Bar	140	
Coffee or tea	10	150 Cal
DINNER		
Frozen Entrée (Appendix D - **page 122**)	290	
"Big-Bowl Salad"	150	
Fresh fruit in season (apple, peach, etc)	70	
Water	0	510 Cal
SNACK		
Popcorn Mini Bag	110	
Coffee or tea	10	120 Cal
		1495 Cal

Day 86 1500 Calorie Meal Plan		
BREAKFAST	Calories	Totals
Cantaloupe (½ medium)	50	
Scrambled egg	80	
Toasted whole-grain bread (1 slice)	70	
Coffee	10	210 Cal
SNACK		
Yogurt (4 oz, non-fat, any flavor)	60	
Coffee or tea	10	70 Cal
LUNCH		
Soup (Appendix B **- page 118**)	170	
String cheese (1 piece, any brand)	80	
Fresh fruit in season (pear, plum, etc)	80	
Coffee or tea	10	340 Cal
SNACK		
Handful unsalted mixed nuts	100	
Coffee or tea	10	110 Cal
DINNER		
Frozen Entrée (Appendix D **- page 122**)	290	
"Big-Bowl Salad"	150	
Whole-grain bread (1 slice)	70	
Fresh fruit in season (apple, peach, etc)	70	
Water with lemon wedge	15	615 Cal
SNACK		
Skinny Cow Ice Cream Sandwich	160	
Coffee or tea	10	170 Cal
		1495 Cal

Day 87 1500 Calorie Meal Plan		
BREAKFAST	Calories	Totals
Cantaloupe (½ medium)	50	
Oatmeal (**½ cup dry) + ½ cup skim milk + 15 raisins**	220	
Coffee	10	280 Cal
SNACK		
Yogurt (4 oz, non-fat, any flavor)	60	
Coffee or tea	10	70 Cal
LUNCH		
Southwest-Style Taco*	270	
Fresh fruit in season (pear, plum, etc)	70	
Coffee or tea	10	350 Cal
* Hot Pockets (wrap)		
SNACK		
Popcorn Mini Bag	110	
Coffee or tea	10	120 Cal
DINNER		
Frozen Entrée (Appendix D **- page 122**)	230	
"Big-Bowl Salad"	150	
Whole-grain bread (1 slice)	70	
Fresh fruit in season (apple, peach, etc)	70	
Water with lemon wedge	15	535 Cal
SNACK		
Kashi TLC Chewy Granola Bar	140	
Coffee or tea	10	150 Cal
		1505 Cal

Day 88 1500 Calorie Meal Plan		
BREAKFAST	Calories	Totals
Cantaloupe (½ medium)	50	
Oatmeal (½ cup dry) + ½ cup skim milk + 15 raisins	220	
Coffee	10	280 Cal
SNACK		
Fresh fruit in season (apple, plum, etc)	70	
Coffee or tea	10	80 Cal
LUNCH		
Frozen Entrée (Appendix D - **page 122**)	290	
Diet soda or water	0	290 Cal
SNACK		
Yogurt (4 oz, non-fat, any flavor)	60	
Coffee or tea	10	70 Cal
DINNER		
Eat Out – Fish dinner		
– Maximum allowable calories	670	670 Cal
SNACK		
100-Calorie Pack Cookies	100	
Coffee or tea	10	110 Cal
		1500 Cal

Day 89 1500 Calorie Meal Plan

BREAKFAST	Calories	Totals
Orange juice (½ cup)	50	
Wheaties (¾ cup) + ½ cup skim milk + ½ banana	190	
Whole-grain toast (1 slice)	70	
Coffee	10	320 Cal
SNACK		
Fresh fruit in season (pear, peach, etc)	70	
Coffee or tea	10	80 Cal
LUNCH		
Soup (Appendix B **- page 118**)	180	
String cheese (1 piece, any brand)	80	
Whole grain bread (1 slice)	70	
Coffee or tea	10	340 Cal
SNACK		
Handful unsalted mixed nuts	100	
Coffee or tea	10	110 Cal
DINNER		
Frozen Entrée (Appendix D **- page 122**)	300	
"Big-Bowl Salad"	150	
Fresh fruit in season (apple, pear, etc)	70	
Hot or iced tea	10	530 Cal
SNACK		
Popcorn Mini Bag	110	
Coffee or tea	10	120 Cal
		1500 Cal

Day 90 1500 Calorie Meal Plan

BREAKFAST	Calories	Totals
Orange juice (½ cup)	50	
Kashi Go Lean Waffles (2)	150	
Morningstar Breakfast Sausage Link	80	
Light Syrup (2 Tbsp)	50	
Coffee	10	340 Cal
SNACK		
Yogurt (4 oz, non-fat, any flavor)	60	
Coffee or tea	10	70 Cal
LUNCH		
Chicken Pot Pie*	230	
Fresh fruit in season (apple, plum, etc)	70	
Diet soda (or water)	0	300 Cal
* Hot Pockets (wrap)		
SNACK		
Handful unsalted mixed nuts	100	
Coffee or tea	10	110 Cal
DINNER		
Frozen Entrée (Appendix D - **page 122**)	200	
"Big-Bowl Salad"	150	
Whole-grain bread (1 slice)	70	
Fresh fruit in season (peach, pear, etc)	70	
Water with lemon wedge	15	515 Cal
SNACK		
Skinny Cow Ice Cream Sandwich	160	
Coffee or tea	10	170 Cal
		1495 Cal

Day 91 1500 Calorie Meal Plan

BREAKFAST	Calories	Totals
Fresh sliced orange	75	
Cheerios (1 cup) + ½ cup skim milk + about 15 raisins	190	
Whole grain toast (1 slice)	70	
Coffee	10	345 Cal
SNACK		
Kashi TLC Chewy Granola Bar	140	
Coffee or tea	10	150 Cal
LUNCH		
Cottage cheese (1 cup low fat)	180	
Fresh fruit in season (apple, plum, etc)	70	
Small whole-grain roll	80	
Coffee or tea	10	340 Cal
SNACK		
Handful unsalted mixed nuts	100	
Coffee or tea	10	110 Cal
DINNER		
Frozen Entrée (Appendix D - **page 122**)	220	
"Big-Bowl Salad"	150	
Whole-grain bread (1 slice)	70	
Water	0	440 Cal
SNACK		
Popcorn Mini Bag	110	
Coffee or tea	10	120 Cal
		1505 Cal

Day 92 1500 Calorie Meal Plan		
BREAKFAST	Calories	Totals
Grapefruit (½)	75	
Scrambled egg	80	
Turkey bacon (1 slice)	35	
Whole-grain toast (1 slice)	70	
Coffee	10	270 Cal
SNACK		
Fresh fruit in season (apple, plum, etc)	70	
Coffee or tea	10	80 Cal
LUNCH		
Salad (3 oz canned tuna, 1 tsp Evoo, onions, celery)	175	
String cheese (1 piece, any brand - 80 Cal max)	80	
Rye bread (1 slice)	70	
Small bunch of grapes	50	
Diet soda or water	0	375 Cal
SNACK		
Yogurt (4 oz, nonfat, any flavor)	60	
Coffee or tea	10	70 Cal
DINNER		
Frozen Entrée (Appendix D - **page 122**)	320	
"Big-Bowl Salad"	150	
Fresh fruit in season (apple, peach, etc)	70	
Water with lemon wedge	15	555 Cal
SNACK		
Dark chocolate (1 oz)	150	
Coffee or tea	10	160 Cal
		1500 Cal

Day 93 1500 Calorie Meal Plan

BREAKFAST	Calories	Totals
Orange juice (½ cup)	50	
Shredded Wheat **(1 cup)** + ½ cup **skim milk** + ½ **banana**	260	
Coffee	10	320 Cal
SNACK		
Nature Valley Crunchy Granola bar	90	90 Cal
LUNCH		
Peanut butter (2 Tbsp) on 2 slices bread	340	
Skim milk (8 oz)	90	
Fresh fruit in season (apple, plum, etc)	70	
Water	0	500 Cal
SNACK		
100-Calorie Pack Cookies	100	
Coffee or tea	10	110 Cal
DINNER		
Frozen Entrée (Appendix D **- page 122**)	190	
"Big-Bowl Salad"	150	
Whole-grain bread (1 slice)	70	
Water	0	410 Cal
SNACK		
Fresh fruit in season (peach, plum, etc)	70	70 Cal
		1500 Cal

Day 94 1500 Calorie Meal Plan		
BREAKFAST	Calories	Totals
Cantaloupe (½ medium)	50	
Oatmeal (½ cup dry) + ½ cup skim milk + 15 raisins	220	
Coffee	10	280 Cal
SNACK		
Fresh fruit in season (apple, peach, etc)	70	
Coffee or tea	10	80 Cal
LUNCH		
Frozen Entrée (Appendix D - **page 122**)	350	
Diet soda or water	0	350 Cal
SNACK		
Yogurt (4 oz, nonfat, any flavor)	60	
Coffee or tea	10	70 Cal
DINNER		
Eat Out – Fish dinner		
– Maximum allowable calories	610	610 Cal
SNACK		
100 Calorie Pack Cookies	100	
Coffee or tea	10	110 Cal
		1500 Cal

Day 95 1500 Calorie Meal Plan

BREAKFAST	Calories	Totals
Fresh sliced orange	75	
Wheaties (¾ cup) + ½ cup skim milk + ½ banana	190	
Whole-grain toast (1 slice)	70	
Coffee	10	345 Cal
SNACK		
Fresh fruit in season (apple, plum, etc)	70	
Coffee or tea	10	80 Cal
LUNCH		
Soup (Appendix B - **page 118**)	100	
String cheese (1 piece, any brand)	80	
Small whole-grain roll	80	
Coffee or tea	10	270 Cal
SNACK		
Handful unsalted mixed nuts	100	
Coffee or tea	10	110 Cal
DINNER		
Frozen Entrée (Appendix D - **page 122**)	350	
"Big-Bowl Salad"	150	
Fresh fruit in season (peach, plum, etc)	70	
Water with lemon wedge	15	565 Cal
SNACK		
Popcorn Mini Bag	110	
Coffee or tea	10	120 Cal
		1490 Cal

Day 96 1500 Calorie Meal Plan

BREAKFAST	Calories	Totals
Orange juice (½ cup)	50	
Wheat Chex (¾ cup) + ½ cup skim milk + ½ banana	250	
Coffee	10	310 Cal
SNACK		
Yogurt (4 oz, nonfat, any flavor)	60	
Coffee or tea	10	70 Cal
LUNCH		
Chicken Broccoli & Cheese*	270	
Fresh fruit in season (peach, plum, etc)	70	
Diet soda or water	0	340 Cal
* Hot Pockets (wrap)		
SNACK		
Handful unsalted mixed nuts	100	
Coffee or tea	10	110 Cal
DINNER		
Frozen Entrée (Appendix D **- page 122**)	220	
"Big-Bowl Salad"	150	
Whole-grain bread (1 slice)	70	
Fresh fruit in season (apple, plum, etc)	70	
Water with lemon wedge	15	525 Cal
SNACK		
Skinny Cow Ice Cream Sandwich	140	
Coffee or tea	10	150 Cal
		1505 Cal

Day 97 1500 Calorie Meal Plan

BREAKFAST	Calories	Totals
Cantaloupe (½ medium)	50	
Scrambled egg	80	
Turkey bacon (2 slices)	70	
Toasted raisin bread (1 slice)	75	
Coffee	10	285 Cal
SNACK		
Yogurt (4 oz, nonfat, any flavor)	60	
Coffee or tea	10	70 Cal
LUNCH		
Soup (Appendix B - **page 118**)	160	
String cheese (1 piece, any brand)	80	
Nature Valley Crunchy Granola bar	90	
Coffee or tea	10	340 Cal
SNACK		
Handful unsalted mixed nuts	100	
Coffee or tea	10	110 Cal
DINNER		
Frozen Entrée (Appendix D - **page 122**)	270	
"Big-Bowl Salad"	150	
Whole-grain bread (1 slice)	70	
Fresh fruit in season (peach, plum, etc)	70	
Water with lemon wedge	15	575 Cal
SNACK		
Popcorn Mini Bag	110	
Coffee or tea	10	120 Cal
		1500 Cal

Day 98 1500 Calorie Meal Plan		
BREAKFAST	Calories	Totals
Grapefruit (½)	75	
Cheerios (1 cup) + ½ cup skim milk + about 15 raisins	190	
Coffee	10	275 Cal
SNACK		
Kashi TLC Chewy Granola Bar	140	
Coffee or tea	10	150 Cal
LUNCH		
Subway 6" (**Ham, Cheese + veggies**)	260	
Fresh fruit in season (apple, plum, etc)	70	
Coffee or tea	10	340 Cal
SNACK		
Handful unsalted mixed nuts	100	
Coffee or tea	10	110 Cal
DINNER		
Frozen Entrée (Appendix D **- page 122**)	200	
"Big-Bowl Salad"	150	
Whole-grain bread (1 slice)	70	
Fresh fruit in season (apple, peach, etc)	70	
Water with lemon wedge	15	505 Cal
SNACK		
Popcorn Mini Bag	110	
Coffee or tea	10	120 Cal
		1500 Cal

Day 99 1500 Calorie Meal Plan

BREAKFAST	Calories	Totals
Grapefruit (½)	75	
Fried egg	80	
Whole-grain toast (1 slice)	70	
Coffee	10	235 Cal
SNACK		
Yogurt (4 oz, nonfat, any flavor)	60	
Coffee or tea	10	70 Cal
LUNCH		
Soup (Appendix B **- page 118**)	180	
Small whole-grain roll	80	
Fresh fruit in season (apple, peach, etc)	70	
Coffee or tea	10	340 Cal
SNACK		
Handful unsalted mixed nuts	100	
Coffee or tea	10	110 Cal
DINNER		
Frozen Entrée (Appendix D **- page 122**)	380	
"Big-Bowl Salad"	150	
Fresh fruit in season (apple, plum, etc)	70	
Diet soda or water	0	580 Cal
SNACK		
Skinny Cow Ice Cream Sandwich	140	
Coffee or tea	10	150 Cal
		1485 Cal

Day 100 1500 Calorie Meal Plan		
BREAKFAST	Calories	Totals
Tomato juice (½ cup)	20	
Shredded Wheat **(1 cup) + ½ cup skim milk + ½ banana**	260	
Coffee	10	290 Cal
SNACK		
Yogurt (4 oz, nonfat, any flavor)	60	
Coffee or tea	10	70 Cal
LUNCH		
Steak, Egg & Cheese*	280	
Fresh fruit in season (apple, peach, etc)	70	
Diet soda (or water)	0	350 Cal
* Hot Pockets (wrap)		
SNACK		
Handful unsalted mixed nuts	100	
Coffee or tea	10	110 Cal
DINNER		
Frozen Entrée (Appendix D **- page 122**)	250	
"Big-Bowl Salad"	150	
Whole-grain bread (1 slice)	70	
Fresh fruit in season (apple, plum, etc)	70	
Water	0	540 Cal
SNACK		
Kashi TLC Chewy Granola Bar	140	140 Cal
		1500 Cal

Appendix A: Shopping Tips

No cooking doesn't mean no preparation! You will probably have to shop once a week. The following should help you prepare your shopping list. First, understand that the problem with basing a meal plan on name-brand food items, such as a particular Lean Cuisine frozen entree, is that the item might not be available where you shop, or it may have been discontinued. What to do? That's where Appendices C and D in this book come in handy. Appendix C lists 19 name-brand soup selections. Appendix D lists more than 100 name-brand frozen meals with their calorie count. Using these lists you should be able to find a substitute for the soup or frozen entree you can't find - a substitute that is based on the same food type, e.g., chicken, fish, or meat, and has the same approximate calorie count.

Substituting Foods

If there is a food listed in the diet you don't like, or perhaps that you forgot to pick up while shopping, you probably can exchange or substitute another food in its place – a technique used by dieticians. Exchanging a food listed in a diet for another food with approximately equal caloric value and nutritional content is the foundation of a successful long-term diet.

Substitution possibilities are almost endless but have to be done carefully. The easiest substitutions are those within the same food group, such as exchanging one vegetable variety for another, or a glass of milk for a cup of yogurt. More sophisticated exchanges cross food groups, for instance replacing 3½ ounces of turkey with a tablespoon of peanut butter spread on a piece of whole wheat bread. Both foods are complete proteins and both contain about 175 Calories. Refer to a good online calorie table to find calorie values. With some understanding and experience, you will be able to substitute foods called for in this diet with equal calorie foods from the same food group.

Another alternative is the following Food Substitution List that suggests substitutions for a variety of food items that appear in the daily meal plans. For example, Day 5 of the diet calls for half a cantaloupe for breakfast. But suppose cantaloupe is not in season, or just doesn't look good, or maybe it's too expensive, or you can't find it at your grocery, from the Food Substitution List you find that you may exchange a ½ cup of orange juice for half cantaloupe – both are in the fruit category and both contain about 50 Calories.

Light Syrup - Use any light syrup (25 Calories per Tbsp)

Big-Bowl Salad - Exchange with unlimited steamed greens (spinach, etc)

Cantaloupe (½) - Use ½ cup Orange juice

Cereal - Exchange with any other whole-grain cereal

Cottage Cheese (1 cup) - Two 8 oz glasses skim milk

Yogurt - Select 6 ounces skim milk

Eggs – Use Egg Beaters

Fresh fruit - ¾ cup canned fruit (no sugar added)

Frozen entrée - Substitute frozen entrée with same calories.

Grapefruit (½) - Choose an orange (medium)

Handful of Nuts - Popcorn Mini Bag

Kashi Chewy Granola Bar - Quaker Chewy Dipps Granola Bar

Kashi Go Lean Waffles - Eggo Nutri-Grain Whole Wheat Frozen Waffles

Hot Pockets Wraps - Lean Pockets Wrap

Morningstar Breakfast Sausage - Any breakfast sausage with comparable calories

String Cheese - Laughing Cow light cheese (2 wedges)

Popcorn - Use handful of mixed nuts

Raisin bread - Plain whole-grain bread

Skinny Cow Ice Cream Sandwich - Skinny Cow Fudge Ice Cream Bar

Soup - Choose any soup with same calorie count

Whole-grain Bread - Vary bread type (whole wheat, rye, etc)

Wine (4 oz) - Instead select grapes (1 cup)

In summary, remember that whenever you encounter a product on this diet, such as "Skinny Cow Ice Cream Sandwich" or "Kashi Go Lean Waffles," that has been discontinued or is out of stock, substitute an equivalent food or desert that is of approximately equal caloric value and nutritional content. In other words substitute a different ice cream product for the "Skinny Cow Ice Cream Sandwich" or a another waffle brand for the "Kashi Go Lean Waffles."

Appendix B: Soup Selections

When the Daily Meal Plan menu specifies soup have only one serving (8 ounces) unless stated otherwise. Note that the listed soups were available in most supermarkets as of 02/14/2020. *These are a canned soup selections.

Soup Description	Calories
Healthy Choice Chicken with Rice	90
Campbell's Tomato	100
Healthy Choice Country Vegetable	100
Progresso Minestrone*	110
Progresso Chickarina*	110
Progresso Italian-Style Wedding*	120
Campbell's Home-Style Light Chicken Corn Chowder*	120
Campbell's Home-Style Chicken Noodle	130
Campbell's Home-Style Butter Nut Squash*	130
Campbell's Healthy Request Vegetable Beef	140
Progresso Lentil*	140
Progresso Green Split Pea*	150
Campbell's Slow Kettle New England Clam Chowder	160
Progresso Macaroni and Bean*	160
Progresso New England Clam Chowder*	170
Progresso Lasagna-Style*	170
Progresso Broccoli Cheese with Bacon*	180
As an alternative, have 2 servings of a 90 Calorie soup	180
Campbell's Chunky Classic Chicken Noodle	190
Amy's Rustic Italian Vegetable*	190
Campbell's Chunky Beef n Cheese*	200
Amy's French Country Vegetable*	210
Campbell's Chunky Sirloin Burger + Vegetables	220
Enjoy two servings of a 110 or 120 Calorie soup	230
Enjoy two servings of a 120 Calorie soup	240

Appendix C: Frozen Food Info

Busy families, singles, older people, and office workers alike enjoy the simplicity and convenience of a frozen meal. Many offices have an employee freezer jammed with all kinds frozen meals, which get zapped in a microwave for a quick, portable, portion-controlled, and relatively inexpensive lunch.

In some cases, frozen may actually be better than fresh, because if you keep fresh fruit and vegetables your fridge for a long time, they lose some of their nutritional value. Whereas, frozen foods are usually processed and packaged within hours of being picked. And the freezing process itself does not destroy nutrients. So buying frozen and then defrosting when you want the fruit or vegetable can actually retain more nutrients.

Storing Frozen Foods

According to the U.S. Department of Agriculture, food stored continuously at 0°F is always safe to eat. Freezing keeps food safe and preserves food for extended periods because it prevents the growth of microorganisms that cause both food spoilage and food-borne illness.

Use an appliance thermometer to monitor your freezer's temperature. If a refrigerator freezing compartment can't maintain 0 °F or if the freezer door is opened frequently, use it for short-term food storage, and eat those foods as soon as possible for best quality. Use a free-standing freezer set at 0 °F or below for long-term storage of frozen foods. Again, keep a thermometer in your freezing compartment or freezer to check the temperature.

Because freezing keeps food safe almost indefinitely, recommended freezer storage times are to preserve quality (taste, etc) of food, not the safety or nutritional value. **The quality of frozen dinners or entrees in a freezer at 0 °F will be maintained for 3 to 4 months**.

If there is a power outage, or if your freezer fails, or if the freezer door is left ajar by mistake, the food may still be safe to use. As long as a freezer with its door ajar continues to run, to cool, the foods should stay safe overnight. If a repairman is on the way or it appears the power will be restored soon, just keep your freezer door closed. A freezer full of food will usually keep about 2 days if the door is kept shut; a half-full freezer will last about a day. The freezing compartment of a refrigerator may not keep foods frozen as long. If the freezer is not full, group packages together to help maintain their low temperature.

During a power failure, you may want to put dry ice, a block or bags of ice in the freezer, or transfer foods to a friend's freezer until power returns. Again, use an appliance thermometer to monitor the temperature. To determine the safety of foods when the power goes on, check their condition and temperature. If food is partly frozen, still has ice crystals, or is as cold as if it were in a refrigerator (40 °F), it is safe to refreeze or use. It's not necessary to cook raw foods before refreezing. **If in doubt discard the food. And always discard frozen food whose temperature has exceeded 40 °F for more than two hours.**

Frozen Food Safety

Increasingly, food giants like ConAgra, Nestlé and others that supply Americans with processed foods concede that they cannot ensure the safety of their food products. Frozen foods pose a particularly serious safety problem because unsuspecting consumers buy frozen foods for their convenience and incorrectly believe that cooking frozen foods is a matter of taste – not safety.

Still the food industry says that extensive outbreaks of food-borne illness are rare, even though it is well-known that most of the millions of cases of food-borne illness every year go unreported or are not traced to the source. For example, each year approximately 40,000 cases of salmonella poisoning are reported in the United States – but perhaps as many as one million cases go unreported. (Salmonella is a type of bacteria most often found in poultry, eggs, unprocessed milk, meat and water.) Recently salmonella pathogens in some frozen meals have sickened thousands of people.

How could this happen? First, the supply chain for ingredients in processed foods – from flour to fruits and vegetables to flavorings – is becoming more complex and global in the drive to keep food costs down. As a result, government and industry officials concede that almost every food ingredient is now a potential carrier of pathogens. A further complication is that a large number of food companies subcontract processing work to save money and don't require suppliers to test for pathogens. In fact, companies often don't even know who is supplying their ingredients.

In addition, many frozen-food manufacturers have stopped cooking their products at high temperatures, a tactic they call the "kill step," which is intended to eliminate any lingering microbes. Frequently this process step turns some of the frozen food ingredients into mush. So, instead the "kill step" has been shifted to consumers. For example, ConAgra has added food safety instructions to its frozen meals, including the Healthy Choice brand. A typical "frozen-food safety" instruction offers this guidance: "Internal temperature needs to reach 165°F as measured by a food thermometer in several spots." Moreover, General Mills, now advises consumers to avoid microwaves altogether and cook their frozen pizzas only in a conventional oven.

Bottom line: To be safe, always cook frozen foods so that the internal temperature reaches 165°F as measured by a good food thermometer.

The Sodium Problem

Sodium and sodium chloride (salt) normally occur in small quantities in many natural foods. People also add salt during food preparation and to the food they eat. But the average sodium intake for American adults is about 3,400 mg daily – more than 1,000 mg higher than the upper limit of 2,400 mg per day recommended by the U.S. Department of Health and Human Services and the Department of Agriculture Dietary Guidelines. (Note that one level teaspoon of salt contains about 2,300 mg of sodium.)

Although sodium plays an important role in your body, many studies have demonstrated that high sodium intake results in excessive water retention which causes blood volume to expand which in turn raises blood pressure. Moreover, some people are more sensitive to the effects of sodium than are others. These sodium-sensitive people retain sodium more easily. If you're in that group, extra sodium in your diet increases your chance of developing high blood pressure, a condition that can lead to cardiovascular and kidney diseases. Individuals who have high blood pressure and who are also salt sensitive are frequently advised to limit their sodium intake even further.

The downside to commercially prepared frozen entrees is that they frequently are loaded with too much salt (sodium). Be aware that, because of the relatively high sodium content of the frozen dinners and microwaveable soups, **the 90-Day No-Cooking Diet may not be appropriate for everyone.**

In fact, you should have a medical checkup before beginning this weight loss diet. And you should let your physician know that the *100-Day No-Cooking Diet* relies to a large degree on commercially processed convenience foods (frozen and microwaveable) – many of which have a relatively high salt (sodium) content.

121

Appendix D: Frozen Entrees

Appendix D lists three popular brands of frozen entrées: Healthy Choice, Lean Cuisine and Smart Ones. The listing is further divided by entrée type: Poultry entrées, Meat entrées, Seafood entrées, Pasta entrées, Pizza and Other entrées. The entire table is arranged from the lowest to highest in calories. Note that the listed frozen entrées were available in most super markets as of 02/14/2020.

Entrée Type	Name	Brand	Calories
Poultry	Tomato Basil Chicken & Spinach	Smart Ones	160
Meat	Steak Portobella	Lean Cuisine	160
Meat	Asian Style Beef & Broccoli	Smart Ones	~~160~~ 170
Poultry	Herb Roasted Chicken	Lean Cuisine	170
Poultry	Slow Roasted Turkey Breast	Smart Ones	170
Poultry	Grilled Chicken Marsala	Healthy Choice	180
Poultry	Creamy Basil Chicken w Broccoli	Smart Ones	~~180~~ 170
Poultry	Garlic Chicken Rolls	Lean Cuisine	180
Meat	Beef Merlot	Healthy Choice	180
Meat	Homestyle Beef Pot Roast	Smart Ones	180
Poultry	Roasted Turkey & Vegetables	Lean Cuisine	190
Poultry	Chicken & Broccoli Alfredo	Healthy Choice	190
Poultry	Chicken & Vegetable Stir Fry	Healthy Choice	190
Other	Broccoli & Cheddar Roast Potato	Smart Ones	190
Poultry	Crustless Chicken Pot Pie	Smart Ones	~~200~~ 190
Poultry	Buffalo Style Chicken	Lean Cuisine	~~200~~ 190
Poultry	Home Style Chicken & Potatoes	Healthy Choice	200
Pasta	Angel Hair Marinara	Smart Ones	200
Poultry	Salisbury Steak	Smart Ones	200
Meat	Roast Beef & Mashed Potatoes	Smart Ones	~~220~~ 200
Pasta	Primavera Pasta	Smart Ones	210
Poultry	Honey Balsamic Chicken	Healthy Choice	210

Entrée Type	Name	Brand	Calories
Pasta	Ravioli Florentine	Smart Ones	210
Poultry	Cajun Style Chicken & Shrimp	Healthy Choice	220
Pasta	Cheese Ravioli Mushroom Sauce	Smart Ones	230
Poultry	Ranchero Chicken Wrap	Smart Ones	230
Poultry	Lemon Herb Chicken Picante	Smart Ones	230
Pasta	Cheese Ravioli Mushroom Sauce	Smart Ones	230
Meat	Meat Loaf with Mashed Potatoes	Lean Cuisine	~~230~~ 240
Seafood	Shrimp Alfredo	Lean Cuisine	~~230~~ 240
Poultry	Chicken Margherita	Smart Ones	~~220~~ 240
Poultry	Grilled Chicken Caesar	Lean Cuisine	240
Poultry	Honey Glazed Turkey & Potatoes	Healthy Choice	240
Pasta	Spicy Penne Arrabbiata	Lean Cuisine	240
Pasta	Four Cheese Cannelloni	Lean Cuisine	~~240~~ 250
Poultry	Creamy Basil Chicken w Tortellini	Lean Cuisine	~~240~~ 250
Pasta	Cheese Ravioli	Lean Cuisine	250
Pasta	Vermont Cheddar Mac & Cheese	Lean Cuisine	250
Pasta	Fettuccini Alfredo	Smart Ones	250
Poultry	Oriental Chicken	Smart Ones	250
Poultry	Fiesta Grilled Chicken	Lean Cuisine	250
Pasta	Chicken Linguini Red Pepper	Healthy Choice	250
Poultry	Golden Roasted Turkey Breast	Healthy Choice	250
Poultry	Chicken Mesquite	Smart Ones	250
Poultry	Chicken Oriental	Smart Ones	250
Poultry	Orange Sesame Chicken	Smart Ones	250
Poultry	Baked Chicken	Lean Cuisine	~~250~~ 260
Poultry	Teriyaki Chicken & Vegetables	Smart Ones	~~250~~ 260
Seafood	Tuna Noodle Casserole	Smart Ones	~~250~~ 270
Pasta	Spaghetti with Meatballs	Lean Cuisine	260
Poultry	Creamy Chicken & Noodles	Healthy Choice	260
Meat	Barbecue Steak with Red Potatoes	Healthy Choice	260

Entrée Type	Name	Brand	Calories
Pasta	Sesame Noodles with Vegetables	Smart Ones	~~260~~ 280
Pasta	Creamy Rigatoni with Chicken	Smart Ones	260
Pasta	Macaroni & Cheese	Smart Ones	260
Pasta	Butternut Squash Ravioli	Lean Cuisine	260
Other	Santa Fe Rice & Beans	Smart Ones	260
Other	Coconut Chickpea Curry	Lean Cuisine	260
Poultry	Glazed Turkey Tenderloins	Lean Cuisine	270
Poultry	Kung Pao Chicken	Healthy Choice	270
Poultry	Chicken Margherita with Balsamic	Healthy Choice	270
Poultry	Chicken Strips & Sweet Potatoes	Smart Ones	270
Pasta	Spaghetti with Meat Sauce	Smart Ones	~~270~~ 280
Meat	Salisbury Steak with Mac & Cheese	Lean Cuisine	~~270~~ 290
Pasta	Penne Rosa	Lean Cuisine	270
Poultry	Turkey Breast & Stuffing	Smart Ones	~~270~~ 280
Pasta	Classic Macaroni & Beef	Lean Cuisine	270
Pasta	Mushroom Mezzaluna Ravioli	Lean Cuisine	270
Pasta	Pasta with Swedish Meatballs	Smart Ones	~~280~~ 290
Other	Asian Pot Stickers	Lean Cuisine	280
Poultry	Sesame Stir Fry with Chicken	Lean Cuisine	280
Poultry	Roasted Turkey Breast	Lean Cuisine	~~280~~ 290
Poultry	Apple Cranberry Chicken	Lean Cuisine	280
Poultry	Chicken Fettuccini Alfredo	Healthy Choice	280
Poultry	Grilled Chicken Marinara	Healthy Choice	280
Poultry	Sweet & Spicy Orange Chicken	Healthy Choice	280
Poultry	Chicken Parmesan	Smart Ones	280
Poultry	Turkey Breast with Stuffing	Smart Ones	280
Meat	Beef & Broccoli	Healthy Choice	280
Meat	Meatball Marinara	Healthy Choice	280
Meat	Beef Teriyaki	Healthy Choice	280
Pasta	Spinach Artichoke Ravioli	Lean Cuisine	280

Entrée Type	Name	Brand	Calories
Pasta	Spinach Artichoke Ravioli	Lean Cuisine	280
Pasta	Linguini with Ricotta & Spinach	Lean Cuisine	280
Poultry	Chicken Fettuccini	Lean Cuisine	~~290~~ 280
Pasta	Spaghetti & Meatballs	Healthy Choice	280
Pasta	Spaghetti with Meat Sauce	Smart Ones	280
Other	Vegetable Fried Rice	Smart Ones	280
Other	Asian Pot Stickers	Lean Cuisine	280
Poultry	Chicken with Almonds	Lean Cuisine	290
Poultry	Chicken with Peanut Sauce	Lean Cuisine	290
Seafood	Shrimp & Angel Hair Pasta	Lean Cuisine	~~280~~ 290
Poultry	Grilled Chicken Pesto w Veggies	Healthy Choice	290
Poultry	General Tso's Spicy Chicken	Healthy Choice	290
Poultry	Pineapple Chicken	Healthy Choice	290
Poultry	Chicken Enchiladas Suiza	Smart Ones	290
Meat	Swedish Meatballs	Lean Cuisine	290
Seafood	Lemon Pepper Fish	Healthy Choice	290
Pasta	Pasta with Swedish Meatballs	Smart Ones	290
Other	Santa Fe Rice & Beans	Smart Ones	290
Pizza	Thin Crust Cheese Pizza	Smart Ones	290
Seafood	Parmesan Crusted Fish	Lean Cuisine	~~290~~ 300
Pasta	Santa Fe-Style Rice & Beans	Lean Cuisine	~~280~~ 300
Poultry	Roasted Turkey & Vegetables	Lean Cuisine	~~290~~ 300
Poultry	Sweet & Sour Chicken	Lean Cuisine	300
Poultry	Crustless Chicken Pot Pie	Healthy Choice	300
Poultry	Sweet Sesame Chicken	Healthy Choice	300
Poultry	Chicken Fettuccini	Smart Ones	300
Poultry	General Tso's Chicken	Smart Ones	300
Meat	Classic Meat Loaf	Healthy Choice	300
Seafood	Tortilla Crusted Fish	Lean Cuisine	~~300~~ 310
Pasta	Tuscan-Style Vegetable Lasagna	Lean Cuisine	~~300~~ 310

Entrée Type	Name	Brand	Calories
Pasta	Broccoli Cheddar Rotini	Lean Cuisine	300
Pasta	Three Cheese Ziti Marinara	Smart Ones	300
Pasta	Lasagna Florentine	Smart Ones	310 300
Seafood	Tortilla Crusted Fish	Lean Cuisine	300 310
Pasta	Tuscan-Style Vegetable Lasagna	Lean Cuisine	300 310
Poultry	Chicken Fried Rice	Lean Cuisine	300 310
Poultry	Orange Chicken	Lean Cuisine	310
Poultry	Chicken Tikka Masala	Lean Cuisine	310
Poultry	Chicken Strips & Fries	Smart Ones	310
Poultry	Chicken Teriyaki	Lean Cuisine	310
Pizza	Thin Crust Pepperoni Pizza	Smart Ones	310
Pasta	Three Cheese Macaroni	Smart Ones	310
Pizza	French Bread Pepperoni Pizza	Lean Cuisine	310
Poultry	Chicken Spinach Mushroom Panini	Lean Cuisine	350 310
Other	Spicy Beef & Bean Enchilada	Lean Cuisine	310
Poultry	Chicken Fried Rice	Healthy Choice	320
Meat	Sweet & Spicy Korean Beef	Lean Cuisine	320
Pizza	Farmers Market Pizza	Lean Cuisine	320
Pizza	Margherita Pizza	Lean Cuisine	320
Poultry	Chicken Carbonara	Lean Cuisine	330
Poultry	Mango Chicken w Coconut Rice	Lean Cuisine	330
Poultry	Country Fried Chicken	Healthy Choice	330
Other	Cheese & Fire-Roasted Tamale	Lean Cuisine	330
Poultry	Chicken Club Panini	Lean Cuisine	350 340
Meat	Philly Style Steak & Cheese Panini	Lean Cuisine	330 350
Poultry	Chicken Parmigiana	Healthy Choice	360
Poultry	Chicken Pecan	Lean Cuisine	320 370
Poultry	Sweet & Sour Chicken	Healthy Choice	390
Pizza	Supreme Pizza	Lean Cuisine	330 390

NoPaperPress eBooks and Paperbacks

100-Day Super Diet-1200 Cal*
100-Day Super Diet-1500 Cal*
100-Day No-Cooking Diet-1200 Cal*
100-Day No-Cooking Diet-1500 Cal*
90-Day Smart Diet-1200 Cal*
90-Day Smart Diet-1500 Cal*
90-Day No-Cooking Diet - 1200 Cal*
90-Day No-Cooking Diet - 1500 Cal*
90-Day Perfect Diet - 1200 Cal*
90-Day Perfect Diet - 1500 Cal*
60-Day Perfect Diet-1200 Cal*
60-Day Perfect Diet-1500 Cal*
50-Day Flex Diet-1200 Cal*
50-Day Flex Diet-1500 Cal*
30-Day Quick Diet - Women*
30-Day Quick Diet for Men*
30-Day No-Cooking Diet*
30-Day Diet for Women - Metric*
30-Day Diet for Men - Metric*
25 Day Easy Diet-1200 Cal*
25 Day Easy Diet-1500 Cal*
25-Day No-Cooking Diet
10-Day Express Diet
10-Day No-Cooking Diet*
7-Day Diet for Women*
7-Day Diet for Men*
7-Day No-Cooking Diets*
90-Day Gluten-Free Diet-1200 Cal*
90-Day Gluten-Free Diet-1500 Cal*
30-Day Gluten-Free Quick Diet*
30-Day Gluten-Free No-Cooking Diet*
7-Day Diet for Women - Metric*
7-Day Diet for Men - Metric
7-Day Gluten-Free Express Diet*
7-Day Gluten-Free No-Cooking Diet*
90-Day Vegetarian Diet-1200 Cal*
90-Day Vegetarian Diet-1500 Cal*
30-Day Vegetarian Diet*
7-Day Vegetarian Diet*
Weight Loss for Women*
Weight Loss for Women - Metric
Weight Loss for Women - UK
Weight Loss for Men*
Maximum Weight Loss - 1200 Cal*
Maximum Weight Loss - 1500 Cal*

Weight Loss for Men - Metric*
Maximum Weight Loss- 1200 Cal*
Maximum Weight Loss- 1500 Cal*
Weight Control - U.S. Edition*
Weight Control - Metric. Edition
Professional Weight Control Women - U.S.
Professional Weight Control Women - Metric
Professional Weight Control Men - U.S.
Professional Weight Control Men - Metric
Weight Maintenance - U.S. Ed*
Weight Maintenance - Metric. Ed*
Weight Maintenance - UK Ed
Weight Loss for Senior Men*
Weight Loss for Senior Women*
Eat Smart - U.S. Edition*
Eat Smart - Metric Edition
30-Day Mediterranean Diet
Exercise Smart - U.S. Edition*
Exercise Smart - Metric Edition
Exercise Smart - UK Edition*
Total Fitness - U.S. Edition
Total Fitness - Metric Edition
Total Fitness - UK Edition
Total Fitness for Women-U.S. Ed*
Total Fitness for Women - Metric
Total Fitness for Women - UK Ed
Total Fitness for Men - U.S. Ed*
Total Fitness for Men- Metric Ed*
Total Fitness for Men - UK Ed
Senior Fitness - U.S. Edition*
Senior Fitness - Metric Edition*
Senior Fitness - UK Edition*
Computer Diet - U.S. Edition*
Computer Diet - Metric Ed*
Reliable Weight Loss - U.S. Ed
101 Weight Loss Tips*
101 Healthy Eating Tips*
101 Lifelong Fitness Tips*
101 Weight Maintenance Tips
101 Weight Loss Recipes
101 GF Weight Loss Recipes
101 Veg Weight Loss Recipes*
30-Day Mediterranean Diet*
90-Day Med Diet - 1200 Cal*
90-Day Med Diet - 1500 Cal*

* These titles are available as both ebooks and paperbacks. Our ebooks are sold by Amazon, Apple, Google, Barnes & Noble and Kobo, but our paperbacks are only sold by Amazon.

Disclaimer

This book offers general meal planning, nutrition and weight control information. It is not a medical manual and the author does not claim to be medically qualified. The material in this book is not intended to be a substitute for medical counseling. Everyone should have a medical checkup before beginning a weight loss program. Moreover, the physician conducting the medical exam should be made aware of and should approve the specific weight control program planned. Additionally, while the author and publisher have made every effort to ensure the accuracy of the information in this book, they make no representations or warranties regarding its accuracy or completeness. Further, neither the author nor publisher assume liability for any medical problems that might result from applying the methods in this book, or for any loss of profit, or any other commercial damages, including but not limited to special, incidental, consequential or other damages, and any such liability is hereby expressly disclaimed.